SIMPLY AUTOPHAGY

How to Leverage Your Body's Natural Intelligence to Reduce Inflammation, Slow Down Aging, Lose Weight Easily through Intermittent Fasting and Other Specific and Targeted Diets!

Josie Kidd

Legal & Disclaimer

Table of Contents

INTRODUCTION 9

CHAPTER 1: WHAT IS AUTOPHAGY? 11

DEFINITION 11

WHY AUTOPHAGY WORKS 12

AUTOPHAGY FOR HEALTH 12

    1. EATING A HIGH FAT, LOW-CARB DIET 12

    2. GO ON A PROTEIN FAST 13

    3. PRACTICE INTERMITTENT FASTING 13

    4. EXERCISE REGULARLY 13

    5. DRINK A LOT OF WATER 14

TYPES OF AUTOPHAGY 14

    1. MACRO-AUTOPHAGY 14

    2. MICRO-AUTOPHAGY 15

    3. CHAPERONE-MEDIATED AUTOPHAGY 16

CHAPTER 2: WAYS TO INITIATE AUTOPHAGY 19

EXERCISE 19

FASTING 20

DECREASE YOUR INTAKE OF CARBOHYDRATES 21

AUTOPHAGY DECREASES THE RATE OF NEURODEGENERATIVE DISEASES 26

AUTOPHAGY CONTROLS INFLAMMATION 26

AUTOPHAGY BOOSTS THE PERFORMANCE OF MUSCLES 26

AUTOPHAGY MAY ENHANCE THE QUALITY OF LIFE 27

AUTOPHAGY BOOSTS THE HEALTH OF THE SKIN........................... 27

AUTOPHAGY ENHANCES YOUR DIGESTIVE HEALTH 27

FIGHT INFECTIOUS DISEASE 28

AUTOPHAGY CAN BOOST A HEALTHY WEIGHT 28

IT REDUCES THE DEATH OF CELLS 29

CHAPTER 3: ANTI-INFLAMMATORY DIET BASICS 31

MOST BENEFICIAL FOODS AND BEST ANTI-INFLAMMATORY
SUPPLEMENTS 33

    BLUEBERRIES 33

    AVOCADO 34

    COENZYME Q10...34

    GINGER 34

    GLUTATHIONE 34

    MAGNESIUM 34

    SALMON...35

    VITAMIN B 35

    VITAMIN D 35

    VITAMIN E..36

    VITAMIN K 36

CHAPTER 4: FOODS THAT REDUCE METABOLIC INFLAMMATION
....37

CHAPTER 5: INTERMITTENT FASTING AND AUTOPHAGY 41

1. THE KETOSIS STATES... 41

2. THE RECYCLING OF CELLS... 41

3. THE 54 HOURS SHIFT 42

INCORPORATING INTERMITTENT FASTING 42

    1. BE PATIENT AND COMPOSED 42

    2. ALWAYS LOOK FOR A GREEN DIET...42

INTO YOUR WORKOUT PLAN... 43

CHAPTER 6: PRECAUTIONS TO TAKE REGARDING AUTOPHAGY AND FASTING...*45*

WHO SHOULD AVOID FASTING 45

WHO NEEDS TO BE CAUTIOUS?.......................................46

CHAPTER 7: INTERMITTENT WATER FASTING 47

CHAPTER 8: COMMON KINDS OF WATER FASTING.................. 49

1. DRY FASTING 49

2. LIQUID FASTING 49

3. JUICE FASTING 49

4. WATER FASTING 49

5. MASTER CLEANSE 50

6. SELECTIVE FASTING 51

CHAPTER 9: WEIGHTLOSS AND WATER FASTING 53

LOSING WEIGHT FOR THE LOOKS 53

LOSING WEIGHT TO GET HEALTHY 54

CHAPTER 10: INTERMITTENT FASTING COULD HELP YOU AGE SLOWLY 57

AUTOPHAGY LOWERS RISK OF NEURODEGENERATIVE DISEASE 58

AUTOPHAGY IMPROVES SKIN HEALTH 58

CHAPTER 11: HOW TO FAST CORRECTLY 59

EXPERIENCE AND DURATION 59

HEALTH...60

NUTRITION AND HYDRATION 60

RELATIONSHIP WITH FOOD...61

CHAPTER 12: AUTOPHAGY, KETOSIS, AND FASTING 63

DOES AUTOPHAGY NEED KETOSIS 63

MEASURE KETONES TO DETERMINE AUTOPHAGY 64

AUTOPHAGY ON KETO 65

ARE KETONES THE BEST FUEL FOR BURNING FAT? 66

HOW KETONES ARE GENERATED 66

WHY YOU NEED TO MAKE KETONES YOUR MAIN FUEL 67

WHAT FOODS TO EAT TO PRODUCE KETONES 67

IS IT POSSIBLE TO INDUCE AUTOPHAGY WITHOUT STARVING
YOURSELF? 68

CHAPTER 13: HYPERTROPHIC GROWTH 69

CHAPTER 14: LONGEVITY AND AUTOPHAGY 73

CHAPTER 15: OXIDATIVE STRESS AND YOUR HORMONES 75

CHAPTER 16: FINDING THE LONG-TERM AND SHORT-TERM
BENEFITS OF AUTOPHAGY 79

IT CAN BE LIFE-SAVING 79

MAY PROMOTE LONGEVITY 79

BETTER METABOLISM 80

REDUCTION OF THE RISK OF NEURODEGENERATIVE DISEASES 80

REGULATES INFLAMMATION 81

HELPS FIGHT INFECTIOUS DISEASES 81

BETTER MUSCLE PERFORMANCE 82

PREVENTS THE ONSET OF CANCER 82

BETTER DIGESTIVE HEALTH 82

BETTER SKIN HEALTH 83

HEALTHY WEIGHT 83

REDUCES APOPTOSIS 83

CHAPTER 17: BENEFITS OF ONE MEAL A DAY 85

KEY BENEFITS..86

WEIGHT LOSS 86

SLEEP 87

RESISTANCE TO ILLNESSES 87

A HEALTHY HEART 87

A HEALTHY GUT.. 88

TACKLES DIABETES 88

REDUCES INFLAMMATION 89

PROMOTES CELL REPAIR 89

IMPROVES MEMORY... 89

REDUCES DEPRESSION 90

CHAPTER 18: FOODS THAT BOOST AUTOPHAGY...................... 91

GINGER...91

GREEN TEA 91

REISHI MUSHROOMS 91

TURMERIC/CURCUMIN 91

EAT PROBIOTICS! 96

CHANGING YOUR EATING HABITS....................................97

DEALING WITH OTHER PEOPLE 98

CHAPTER 19: CIRCADIAN RHYTHMS AND AUTOPHAGY 101

CHAPTER 20: SLEEP OPTIMIZATION................................... 103

CONCLUSION 107

INTRODUCTION

Autophagy protects bone density and muscle mass. The mineral intake that you get after having autophagy can protect your bone density. The bones need certain minerals that are used to cure the excessive number of hurdles one gets while running. The minerals are given by autophagy, and you are able to get a stronger bone for life. If you are a bodybuilder and want to reap the benefits of the bone, then you have to accumulate more autophagy in you that can be very beneficial for you. The muscle mass can be secured in an acute manner if you tend to get more and more almonds and other alkaline dietaries. You have to be very lenient when you are having autophagy because the benefit of autophagy, such as muscle muscle mass and bone density, will be instrumental for you. Just always look at the bright side of the diet, and you will feel very productive while you do it.

In today's world, tensions are like a haunting disease that wants to remain at your back for no reason. Everywhere you go, you get a tertiary level of tension. There is the tension of graduating, the tension of succeeding in life, the tension of getting a job, and the tension of whatnot. You believe that tension can be very successive for you, but in the latter, it turns out to be adverse. Scientists have claimed many medical drugs for their cure, but the only reasonable cure is the use of an alkaline diet. The enzymes that you get through vegetables lower the risk of your hyper blood tension, and then you can achieve all the relish of your lifestyle in no time. Also, your blood level starts to resonate with full capacity, and you will feel like a superman every place you go, therefore, hypertension and tensed matters get an upper hand of resolution when you get to know the prospect of an alkaline diet.

Over time, our cells produce by-products and waste from the hard work that they are constantly doing. This microscopic bio-waste is collected in the cell, like an overflowing trash can. This happens when we eat too many sugars and carbohydrates, changing our insulin absorption and affecting our whole system's ability to function properly. When the cells are running slow because the waste is building up on account of a poor diet, lack of exercise, and our over-consumption of food daily, slowly over time, we begin to see the results: cancer, diabetes, inflammatory disease, cardiovascular disease, and rapid aging.

Our bodies are intelligent and know how to clean house and heal, especially if we create the right conditions for this process to occur. Autophagy is a self-healing mechanism at the cellular level that, when achieved, can change the health of your whole life.

CHAPTER 1: WHAT IS AUTOPHAGY?

This chapter will deal with the definition, the working of autophagy, the types of autophagy, and the usage of autophagy in the coming time. This chapter will also include the various formations of autophagy through which the people's way is moved forward in the direction. The contextualization of the book is as follows:

DEFINITION

According to Doctor Priya Khorana, the process of autophagy means the exit of food through the stomach, and it makes the metabolism look very clean. The cells that are used in this process are easily removed during this process, and later there is the rejuvenation of newer cells for healthy growth for humans. Auto means self, and the word phagy means eating. Therefore, autophagy means that the body will eat automatically, and with the passage of time, the old food will be removed.

By some authors, it is also related to self-devouring. This is the beneficial omen for your body and the process of self-devouring. The body cells are easily extinguished from the body thoroughly. The process of cellular repair also takes place in this context, and the over-all body metabolism reaches its zeal. Thus, the use of cellular repair will make the body look better in the coming. The process of autophagy is a revolutionary self-preserving mechanism that helps in the elimination of carbon-related diseases in the human body.

For some, the definition is also contextualized as the process through which the cells of the body easily function in a better manner. There is also the removal of debris. It is referred to as the process of recycling and removing at the same time. The prolific medical scientist referred to it as the way of resetting your body, and the body aims to reach the better part of life. It is also a promotion of better toxin-related concepts of the body, and it will amplify the metabolism of the body in a perpetual manner.

WHY AUTOPHAGY WORKS

There is an ancient saying that the body will work if led with a proper mind. The use of autophagy helps to instill a proper mode of management for the people through which the persons are able to lead a happy life. The working of autophagy is also productive because it is able to give marvelous and potential results to the human body. It creates the possibility and creation of better cells that are quite great in their number, and they are able to curb strong measurements of disease prevention in them. There are many other benefits of it through which the body is able to receive better quality digestion and heat of hydration. There are numerous working mechanisms that are cultivated in the body through the use of autophagy. Since the use of autophagy brings about better changes in the human body, therefore, the use of autophagy works in the coming time, and it is much effective for the use of the human body.

AUTOPHAGY FOR HEALTH

There are five important ways through which autophagy works for the construction of health for the students and civilians. These ways help to restore the health factor for autophagy constructively.

1. EATING A HIGH FAT, LOW-CARB DIET

The eating of a high-fat triggers autophagy in the body. The use of high fat and its gestation ultimately exits some cells from the body through which the people are able to have a better understanding of the body in their dimension. The low carb diet will make your suit for autophagy as the process of elimination of cells will be random in the body, and the person will be able to give more value to its body. So, the intake of high fat will make the body have more leniency in it, and with the passage of time, the body will get rid of all the cells that make the body look pale and obstructive in the coming time.

2. GO ON A PROTEIN FAST

The autophagy will be helpful for the protein fast. Because in this fast you will be able to do a lot of mass exemption from the body. During the fast of the body, the people will be able to have a better comprehension of the body through which the protein of the body will go away, and the body will be given a better way of creating proteins in the coming time. Therefore, going on a protein fast will help to make the body a much better and more regulatory space.

3. PRACTICE INTERMITTENT FASTING

The concept of intermittent fasting is that the body has to take a lot of proteins from the human body, and there is a regular break from eating and drinking. There are time intervals through which the body is able to garner more food and water in the body. This time can be used to make the body look better and productive in the coming time. The use of strong fasting can make the body relax and have a sustainable work in the coming. So, if you want to attain a benefit from autophagy for health, then practice intermittent fasting.

4. EXERCISE REGULARLY

Exercising regularly can also initiate a fast rate of autophagy for you. Exercise helps to reduce fats allowing for more proteins to actually work in the body. The working of the body helps to maintain a strong pH value of the system, and the body is able to foment a healthier metabolism. This is a concept through which the autophagy of the body functions in a better way, and with the passage of time, autophagy tends to be sustainable in a better function.

5. DRINK A LOT OF WATER

Drinking a lot of water also helps you to maintain a stable metabolism of yourself through which you are able to have a yielding understanding of things around. Drinking a lot of water makes the ph value system aware of all the things happening around, and with the passage of time, the body is able to make healthier changes in the coming time. Drinking a lot of water will keep the diet clean and healthy, and it will make your body fit for any changes coming in the contemporary. Therefore, drinking a lot of water is crucial for you to maintain an autophagy state.

TYPES OF AUTOPHAGY

There are three types of autophagy. One is the macro-autophagy, micro-autophagy, and chaperone-mediated autophagy.

1. MACRO-AUTOPHAGY

Macro-autophagy is a type of autophagy in which the degradation of organelles occurs. It is a matured vesicle process. It is strongly recommended for the homeostasis process, in which the persons belonging to various paths and parallels are identified in the human being for a perpetual state of mind. The use of macro-autophagy can be illustrated in many ways of the world. The uses are very much in use these days. The use of microautophagy can be related to many uses like the cure of brain diseases and brain coverages. The use of macroautophagy has many abilities embedded in it. It can be used to treat neurodegenerative diseases in people. The disease-linked aggresomes can be used in many uses to make the fossils and the human platelets working in a better way. The macroautophagy can also be constructed in many ways possible for the people coming forward. Therefore, Macroautophagy is the branch of autophagy, which deals with the process of clearing the established fats in the body.

2. MICRO-AUTOPHAGY

The construct of microautophagy is different from two types of autophagy that are macro and chaperone-mediated autophagy. These autophagias help the micro people and the lysosomal action to be easily overridden by the people and the body state. This practice is adopted by many people abroad, and it can also be found with many people and other doctors to be precisely relevant. This practice is very important for the functioning of cells, and it helps to give more emphasis to the extermination of diseases in the coming time. Cytoplasmic material is trapped in the cells of the people, and the people are able to manifest the uses of autophagy properly. This process is also used for nitrogen deprivation, and it can lead to strong illustrations of people effectively. There are three special cases of microautophagy. Micro hexalogy, piecemeal microautophagy, and microautophagy of the nucleus. These phages make the body of the human being emerged from the ashes.

There are very important functions of micro-autophagy. There are used for nutrient recycling. This is done for the degradation of lipids. It regulates the composition of the vacuolar membrane. There are many mechanisms of glycogen in it. The pathway that comes through micro-autophagy helps to create a link with the multivesicular bodies, endocytic, membrane proteins, and the use of strong organelle size. There is also non-selective micro-autophagy in this regard. There is membrane invagination, vesicle formation, vesicle expansion, vesicle degradation, and selective micro-autophagy. These invaginations help to create a better formation of body cells for the persons coming forward, and with the passage of time, the body is able to eat all the fats and vitamins of the structure effectively. This practice is of strong use and pertinence and can be regarded effectively in the coming time.

The process of selective micro-autophagy can be observed in all types of eukaryotic cells. On the other hand, this is also commonly observed in yeast cells. Therefore, micro-autophagy helps to create a cluster of better engines for the coming community.

3. CHAPERONE-MEDIATED AUTOPHAGY

This chaperone-mediated autophagy helps to give more ideas to the process of autophagy. This is referring to the selection of chaperone dependent selection. The selection of soluble proteins is taken into account. The cytosolic proteins are targeted to lysosomes and are directly related to the concept of lysosome membrane without the requirement of the formation of additional values. The proteins that want to make the structure of CMA are cytosolic proteins and proteins from other compartments. There are some compartments that discuss the nature of CMA, and they are worthy of being discussed here. These are the compartments that tend to make the working of the cells more functional and linear in their working. There is a selectivity of proteins, and the proteins are able to make the manufacture of the engine more compatible. The CMA can be of many uses and regards of the people, and the people are able to blend with the work coherently.

The proteins that participate in the CMA are more likely to be engulfed by the main cell of the body. First there is the degradation of cells, there is the presence of cytosolic protein in the making, there is the formation of amino acid in work, there is lysosome-associated work of the protein type A in the formation, there is a receptor for the membrane of the formation of the work, the two isoforms are found in the cells of the body through which one has to trade genes to the people coming ahead, there are substrates that deal with the process of working for the people and then there are translocation purposes that make the deal of CMA more workable. There is an artificial use of people that do not cater properly to the formation of the work, and with the passage of time, there is a better comprehension thing coming forward.

The matter comes to the people of the formation in a close manner, and this thing helps to bind the CMA more effectively for the people.

Therefore, the use of a close manner can be sorted out more periodically in the coming time. There are some limitations to the CMA process. One is the binding of the substrate of the people coming forward, and with the passage of time, the CMA tends to be more linear with time. There are some levels of constraints to the process of CMA as well. With the passage of time, the CMA tends to devolve, and if one wants to maintain a proper outlook of CMA, then there need to be some limitations. The levels of CMA are easily utilized, and they are made under some uncertainties for the people. The people in these uncertainties are not able to proceed with CMA, and hence, they are able to come stringently ahead.

These are three types of autophagias discussed above in an effective manner.

Once you are able to identify the process by understanding the different ways autophagy can occur inside the cell, you can picture the process and connect the dots with why you might want to activate autophagy in your body. If you have never fasted, experienced ketosis through your food intake, or had any kind of exercise routine, then you are likely walking around with some very cluttered cells that need some serious cleanup. Autophagy is always happening on some level; however, when you are not creating circumstances to help it occur optimally, then it is only working at a moderate to low level of efficiency. There are many ways that initiating autophagy can improve your health and prevent serious or chronic health conditions later in life.

Even though self-degradation occurs in nearly every organism's cells as a survival mechanism, from yeast to humans, there are three different ways in which the cell delivers what it longer needs to the degradation vesicle – the lysosome. These can be distinguished depending on how the cell forms the lysosome, the number of steps required, and the cargo contained in the vesicles.

Most of the cellular waste is eliminated through macroautophagy, which has long been considered the default pathway and by far the most studied. During macroautophagy, cells use their own membranes to form two types of vesicles: one called autophagosome, which captures any product, and the lysosome, containing enzymes that help speed up the recycling process. Microautophagy is a more straight-forward way to achieve the same result, however, it's not molecule-specific: any substance can be removed from the cell's interior and directly delivered to the lysosome. Recently, studies described a subtype of microautophagy that helps the cell integrate proteins produced at the endoplasmic reticulum, proving that autophagy is not an exclusively catabolic mechanism.

On the opposite end of the spectrum, we have CHAPERONE-MEDIATED AUTOPHAGY, that only targets protein into the lysosome. Each protein is assigned to a signaling molecule that is then recognized by chaperones included in the degradation of the vesicle membranes. In some cases, chaperones can also recognize transcription factors, proteasomes, and proteins involved in cellular transportation systems. For this to happen, proteins must present a very specific structural pattern, the KFERQ motif. Without this motif, chaperone-mediated autophagy cannot progress normally, as it's essential for the uptake and unfolding process that occurs at the lysosome.

CHAPTER 2: WAYS TO INITIATE AUTOPHAGY

You may be on board with the idea of having your cells eat each other, but are probably now wondering how you would go about doing it. Or more accurately, how you would trigger your body to kick start this process for you. The good news is that autophagy is a response to stress. This means that when you stress your body in certain ways, the process is triggered. But not all stress will do the trick. When you add a little bit extra stress to your body, the self-consumption process is elevated. This added stress can be uncomfortable at the moment, but the idea is that this little bit of extra stress can lead to incredible, long-term joy. Adding more stress in a controlled manner can result in amazing benefits to your body. There are three primary ways to induce your autophagy process; exercise, fasting, and decrease your carbohydrate intake significantly.

EXERCISE

You have probably heard for a long time now that diet and exercise are the keys to a long and healthy life. This is no different, and the science to back up this is here for you in the first and second chapters. Exercise stresses your body at the moment. This is why people have pains after a hard workout, grunt when it is challenging, and sweat. When your muscles work hard, they get little tears in them that need to be repaired. Your body responds to these tears quickly, and while repairing the damage you just did, the body makes the muscle stronger so it can resist any future "damage" you might inflict upon it. You may not think of exercising as a way to clean out your cellular buildup of toxins, but it's one of the most common and popular ways to renew your cells. This helps explain why you feel so fresh and rejuvenated after a good, hard workout.

In one study on mice with highlighted autophagosomes, the researchers found that after they ran on a treadmill for 30 minutes their autophagy process was dramatically increased. An autophagosome is a resulting structure in the autophagy process. It forms around the damaged or toxic part of the cell and removes it to be disposed of, leaving behind the healthy parts of the cell. The increase in exercise provided evidence that these became more efficient and frequent than when the mice for less active. And it did not just increase the rate of autophagy while exercising! The increased rate of self-consumption continued for 80 minutes after stopping exercising. While there are no concrete studies or information regarding how much or how often a human should exercise to increase autophagy, it is clear the relationship exists in humans as well. Dr. Daniel Klionsky, a University of Michigan cellular biologist, explains that it is hard to determine the level of exercise a human must undergo to trigger their autophagy process, but there are so many clear benefits to exercise that no matter what you do, it will help support your body on some level. The best assumption to make in this case is to engage in more intense exercise regimens a few times a week for the best results. This is for general health benefits, but will also be the best amount of controlled stress on your body to trigger your autophagy.

FASTING

Cleanses that introduce any form of food or drink besides water into the body will actually prevent the trigger of autophagy, not allowing the body to effectively cleanse itself of toxins, as desired on a cleanse. Instead, simply skipping a meal or two or three can be the best stress on the body that triggers autophagy, offering a true cleanse. Your body will probably not like it at the moment, but the benefits will be something it will enjoy for a long time. Research has shown, over and over again, that engaging in an occasional fast can help you lower risks of various illnesses like heart disease and diabetes. The reason for these benefits that medical professionals and scientists claim is because of autophagy.

There are several studies that have been published that specifically look at fasting, autophagy, and brain health. It is clear there is a distinct connection between lowering the risk of developing a neurodegenerative disease, like Parkinson's disease or Alzheimer's disease, when you engage in short-term fasts. Other studies reveal that intermittent fasts help support proper brain function, brain structure, and neuroplasticity. This is what helps your brain learn new information easier. While this information is exciting, it is not completely clear if autophagy is the reason, and most of these studies are conducted on animals. While the benefits are promising, they are not always applicable to human subjects.

There are a variety of adaptations for intermittent fasting, and it is something that can fit into almost anyone's life because of this. You can choose to abstain from eating food anywhere between 12 to 36 hours in a stretch, always drinking a lot of water during the fast. You can also engage in moderate to light physical activity during this time to help your body upregulate the results, but it is not typically advisable to engage in intense workouts during a fasting period. In addition, you can choose to fast only during certain times of the year, a certain day of the month, or one or more days a week.

DECREASE YOUR INTAKE OF CARBOHYDRATES

Fasting on a regular basis can be a challenge for many people, especially if you are used to constantly eating. In addition, this is contradictory to a lot of popular advice available now, encouraging people to eat little meals consistently throughout the day to boost metabolism. What research has shown, however, is that eating constantly does not keep your metabolism and hunger "satisfied" but rather creates a constant "hunger" hormone that keeps you wanting to eat and eat. Instead, when you fast, you learn the difference between true hunger and a triggered response at the time you normally eat a meal. You break your body of these habits and encourage it to focus on your cellular repair and fat-fuel burning instead. If you are having trouble getting into an intermittent fasting schedule, you can mimic the benefits in another way by decreasing your intake of carbohydrates.

This similar process is called ketosis. A lot of people who work out regularly or are looking to improve their long-term health and well-being have been turning to this type of eating regimen. The concept aims to significantly reduce the carbs that are consumed, so your body must use the fat for fuel instead of injected glucose from the conversion of the carbs. When your body enters into ketosis, it mirrors a lot of the same changes to your metabolism that autophagy offers. You get to enjoy the benefits of fasting without having to complete fast. In addition to the similar benefits to your metabolism, ketosis has been shown to help you maintain healthy body weight, protect your muscle mass, prevent and fight tumors, lower your risk of type-2 diabetes, minimize the risk of neurological diseases, and treat some brain disorders, like epilepsy. For example, in one recent study, more than 50% of the children with epilepsy that followed this diet experienced more than half the frequency of seizures than their peers not following the diet.

In addition to removing a lot of the carbs, you increase your intake of healthy fat. Most of your calories, up to 70%, come from fat on the Keto diet. This means eating a lot of meat, avocado, peanut butter, to name a few. Protein is up to 30% of your daily caloric intake. If you have room for carbs, you need to keep them to less than 50 grams every day. This is an extreme diet that many people get used to over time. If you can, being with a mix of fat/protein/carbs with your carb intake not exceeding 30% of your daily caloric intake and work back from there. Some find this regimen of eating more challenging than fasting, so it is wise to look into and try out what method works best for you in triggering your autophagy response.

If you are still looking at these three primary methods for triggering autophagy and wondering if there are other, easier ways, you will be discouraged to find that there are none. There will be a lot of money when researchers find a way to trigger autophagy or mimic it in a synthetic form like a pill, and it is being researched and considered now, but this is a long way off. Until the process is better understood, it is not possible to chemically induce the process in a human body. It is also unwise to turn to synthetic and chemical methods to avoid dieting and exercise for your well-being. It is also important to note that there are anti-epilepsy drugs being developed to mirror the state of ketosis in the body. If those become available, it is probable that people will begin taking them to mimic autophagy in the body instead of approaching it through traditional diet and exercise methods.

Keep in mind that the process of ketosis in the body is complex, as the process of autophagy. The idea that a single pill can mimic this entire, intricate, and complex process is unrealistic. The stress required to enter ketosis, for example, may be an integral part of the process. This means you will need to still exert effort and energy to get the pill to work in any form. It is also likely that the pill will only encourage one or two of the benefits of ketosis for a person suffering from epilepsy and not target any other benefits of ketosis. Yes, the three methods of activating autophagy and ketosis listed above all require effort, and it is important to also remember that you do not need to do each of them every day to get the results and benefits. Just a couple of hours a week or month can do the trick for supporting your cellular health.

Finally, there is a lot of published research available to show the indication of the various benefits of autophagy as well as how to activate it in a healthy way. The little bit of short-term and controlled stress can lead to controlled and systematic self-destruction so you can end up living a longer, healthier life. It is an ancient survival process that is designed to help the body in times of stress, like when your ancestors had to go days between meals that they hunted to feed themselves and their family. Starvation and physical exertion have the ability to kill you, but over millions of years, human bodies have evolved to turn those "bad" situations into something that can actually help you.

The molecular nature of autophagy was first discovered in budding yeast Saccharomyces cerevisiae as a model structure, functioning in all eukaryotic organisms but not in prokaryotes. Autophagic activity is necessary for the improvement of cellular homeostasis and energy balance.

A lot of evidence relates to malfunctions in autophagic processes to most clinically applicable diseases, including neurodegeneration, autoimmunity, cardiovascular disease, and diabetes. The creation of autophagy-focused therapies will rely on an extensive understanding of the benefits, and possible results, of changing autophagic activity.

Different forms of autophagy have been differentiated using the cargo is degraded. The most extensively researched type of autophagy –macro-autophagy reduces huge sizes of the cytoplasm and cellular organelles. Also, the selection of individual substrate classes, cytoplasmic organelles, protein aggregates, and bacteria requires special adaptors that identify the cargo and focuses on the autophagosomes membrane. Other types of autophagy comprise macroautophagy, which requires the direct surrounding of cytoplasmic material through inward folding of the lysosomal membrane, and chaperone-mediated autophagy (CMA).

While autophagy is a degradative channel, it also takes part in biosynthetic and secretory processes. Since autophagy plays a big role in most essential cellular functions. It is not a surprise that autophagic dysfunction is related to multiple forms of human diseases.

Misfolded proteins have a tendency to create insoluble compounds that are dangerous to the cells. To solve this problem, the cells rely on autophagy.

Why autophagy is special, the response depends on the degree of flexibility of autophagosomes size and selection of cargo. Autophagy can support degradation en masse for numerous and different forms of substrates allowing cells to quickly and effectively build up recycled basic building materials in the face of a broad type of nutritional deficiencies.

Besides this, autophagy is the only medium that is capable of degrading whole organelles, randomly or in a targeted style. This is a critical procedure for regulating homeostasis in the complex landscape of the eukaryotic cell. This process authenticates a quality control mechanism that is important for counteracting the negative effects of aging. Autophagy refers to a dynamic, multi-step process that consists of autophagosomes development, depletion of the autophagic substrate, and autolysosome development. The development of autophagosomes, a thin membrane vesicle that surrounds cytosolic components into lysosomes for depletion and recycling, represents autophagy. During the time of autophagy stimulation, the cytoplasmic type of microtubule-related protein 1 light chain LC3 is lipidated and admitted to the autophagosomes. LC3 II, which is the lipidated type of LC3, is connected to the autophagosome membrane, which makes LC3 conversion a must for autophagosome development. The popularly used assay for tracking autophagic flux is the turnover of LCB, which measures the content using autophagic flux. But this method is time-consuming and labor intensive, and the results are usually in different experimental settings and difficult to interpret. Understanding the need for a strong method to highlight autophagic compartments with little straining of endosomes and lysosomes is a critical approach for tracking autophagy and approximating the autophagic flux in active cells.

Now, let us examine the important benefits of autophagy in detail.

Although "self-eating" may look like a bad idea, it can be a source of youth and for your cells to regenerate. The phrase "autophagy" is a state for our cells to switch to repair damage and heal. This healing state is stimulated when we need to fight infection, save energy, and repair damage. Read on to discover why autophagy matters in your life.

AUTOPHAGY DECREASES THE RATE OF NEURODEGENERATIVE DISEASES

A lot of brain aging diseases take a lot of time to develop because they are the outcome of proteins in and around your brain cells that don't work right. Autophagy assists cells in cleaning up the proteins that don't do their work, and they are less likely to add. For example, autophagy removes amyloid in Alzheimer's disease and a-synuclein in Parkinson's disease. There is an explanation why dementia is believed to be at par with diabetes: the constant high blood sugar controls autophagy from activating, making it difficult to prevent these cells from clutter.

AUTOPHAGY CONTROLS INFLAMMATION

Autophagy stimulates a "Goldilocks" degree of inflammation by quelling the immune response you require. Autophagy can boost inflammation when an invader is available by stimulating the immune system to attack. In most cases, autophagy reduces inflammation from your immune response by halting the signals that trigger it.

AUTOPHAGY BOOSTS THE PERFORMANCE OF MUSCLES

As you build microtears and inflame muscles while exercising, the muscles need repair. The demand for energy increases. Your muscle cells will respond to this by getting into autophagy to decrease the energy needed to use the muscle and enhance the balance of energy to lower the risk of future damage.

AUTOPHAGY MAY ENHANCE THE QUALITY OF LIFE

The advantages of anti-aging may appear to be too good to be true, but the truth is more than the outer layer of the skin. Since the 1950s, scientists have been researching the process of autophagy, but recent studies have disclosed more about how it enhances cellular health. Rather than consuming new nutrients, the cells undergo autophagy to recycle the damaged parts they have, eliminate toxic material and fix themselves up. When your cells repair on their own, they work better, and they can work like younger cells. You may have noticed that some people have a very separate chronological and biological age. The degree of damage a body has taken and how it has managed to repair plays a big role in these differences.

AUTOPHAGY BOOSTS THE HEALTH OF THE SKIN

The cells that you expose to the world experience a lot of damage from air pollution, cold, chemicals, heat, humidity changes, and physical damage. That is the reason why it doesn't appear worse for wear. Once the cells of your skin hold toxins and damage, they start to age in place. Although your body creates new cells, autophagy can assist repair the current ones so that you glow well. Skin cells fight bacteria that may destroy the body, so it is important to support them as they clean the clutter.

AUTOPHAGY ENHANCES YOUR DIGESTIVE HEALTH

The cells inside your gastrointestinal tract are always triggered to function. In fact, a large percentage of your feces are your cells. With the help of autophagy, your digestive cells can repair and restore, clean themselves of junk, and activate the immune system as required. Since a chronic immune system within the gut can exhaust and inflame your bowels, an opportunity to repair, rest, and recover is crucial to your health. Stimulate autophagy using a schedule that supports an extended overnight fast, and you can offer your gut space it requires to heal.

FIGHT INFECTIOUS DISEASE

Autophagy can help accept an immune response when required. Next, the process of autophagy can eliminate specific microbes directly from the inside cells like Mycobacterium tuberculosis, or even viruses like HIV. Autophagy can still eliminate the toxins generated by infections, which is necessary for foodborne illness.

AUTOPHAGY CAN BOOST A HEALTHY WEIGHT

Below are unique benefits of autophagy that create a healthy body:

- **Autophagy demands fat-burning to be turned on but spares protein. On a very long fast, you will lose a protein mass, but in short fasting periods, you can stimulate autophagy, spare protein, burn fat, and receive all the benefits of a leaner and fitter you.**

- **Autophagy suppresses unnecessary inflammation. Chronic inflammation increases insulin, resulting in more weight storage-and less inflammation assist in decreasing the percentage of insulin.**

- **Autophagy decreases toxins inside the cell body. As long as you can remove toxins, they are less likely to require fat cells to store them.**

- **Autophagy permits metabolic efficiency by repairing the sections of cells that make and package proteins and synthesis energy, which is important when cells require to shift to fat-burning for energy.**

IT REDUCES THE DEATH OF CELLS

Compared to cell death, the death of a cell is messy and builds garbage to clean up. Your body awakens inflammation to perform the clean –up. The higher the percentage of cells that repair themselves before they are damaged beyond repair, the less effort your body put into cleaning old cells and regenerating new ones. Minimal inflation is involved in regenerating tissues. You can make use of this energy to substitute cells that require continuous renewal, such as digestive cells. Although there are specific cells that need to be turned over a lot, not all cells need this. A lot of repair with minimal cleanup is a huge mix of success. While there are a lot of health benefits you can gain, it is a repair response to stress.

As we close on this chapter, autophagy performs two main roles. First, it removes damaging materials and foreign invaders. Secondly, it synthesizes cellular materials for energy during times of starvation. Improper control of autophagy is a big factor for numerous diseases like diabetes, autoimmune diseases, cancer, and infections. Not only does it eliminate damaged materials-it also activates senescence and enhances the cell present antigens on its surface. Researchers have started to establish autophagy as a critical process in both pathology and physiology.

CHAPTER 3: ANTI-INFLAMMATORY DIET BASICS

There are many forms of inflammation in the body. Some can be temporary, some chronic. Some forms that start as temporary may turn into a chronic condition. Along with multiple forms of inflammatory conditions, there are also as many opinions or more on how to treat them, bring down discomfort levels, or even just generally work to make you feel better.

So how do you pick and choose as to what is the best way for you to address whatever inflammatory condition you or a loved one may be experiencing? As with any medical condition, the first thing to do is to discuss it with your doctor. Even for those who prefer not to follow a more allopathic route (via western M.D., etc. solutions), let's face it—at the very least, our medical practitioners have worked and studied very hard at finding the various ways to make us feel better. Dr. Google is not always going to have the best answers for us or may have too many conflicting and confusing answers, leaving us lost to wade through a myriad of information mingled with misinformation.

What does this mean for those who want to be proactive in their health and supplement other treatments with additional avenues to help make themselves feel better? It means that you need to learn more about the health condition with which you are facing, how it affects you on different levels, and what additional options might be available to you.

Luckily, there are many aspects of anti-inflammatory conditions that can be addressed in a beneficial manner with a few simple lifestyle changes. This is not to say that these are cures, but rather, they can be beneficial toward pain reduction and ease of living. In the case of this guide, the discussion will be focused on not only the dietary aspects of the equation, but also as a well-rounded aspect from which you can attack your chronic issues from all sides. Diet can be looked at as more than just the food you put into your body. It is the nourishment provided to the body, something you experience repeatedly. Repetition creates habits. When dealing with chronic inflammation, it is necessary to break old, bad habits that increase the inflammation and replace them with a habitual diet of new and good habits that help you to feel better!

While there are some very basic steps that will help many or even most people, the first understanding you need in order to create fewer frustrations in any pursuit of lifestyle changes is that not everything will work for everyone. You could even be one of those people for whom nothing seems to work. It can happen. The closer look that you take at how your body actually *does* work in conjunction with the diagnosis for the condition you are facing, the more readily you stand the chance of finding what *does* work for you.

Sometimes the search for relief means a series of trials and errors. It is how research is done. Regardless of how frustrating this can be, it can help to take a positive outlook. You may not always find the answer you seek, but what you may find is what doesn't work for you. It is a process of elimination that can help in your search for a better quality of life. So don't get discouraged. Consider every step as a step in a positive direction. Learning what doesn't work for you can be just as important as what does. It will help you tailor your solutions specifically to you and your health and well-being.

As human beings with a myriad of genetic make-ups, backgrounds, areas, and conditions under which we have been raised or currently live, additional and/or multiple medical conditions, along with so many other influencing factors, we are each unique. How could it be any different in what will and will not work to make you feel better?

The pages to follow within this guide are designed to help you better understand how inflammatory conditions affect your overall body and health, why things generally do and do not work to make you feel better, and overall, to help you better understand your own body so, in turn, you can find what helps to make your body *feel* better.

As you step through the basics on the pages within this guide, take the time to learn about you. No one source is going to be the definitive "go-to" for everyone, but hopefully, you will find something to take away and make your journey on your way back to feel better, more positive and pleasant experience.

MOST BENEFICIAL FOODS AND BEST ANTI-INFLAMMATORY SUPPLEMENTS

Many conditions can be traced back to inflammation. Joint pain, autoimmune disorders, irritable bowel syndrome (IBS), mood imbalances, acne, and eczema are just a few conditions that can be linked back to inflammation. Once the origin of inflammation is identified, an anti-inflammatory diet can help ease symptoms, and certain foods and supplements can help lessen the inflammation in your body. In this chapter, we'll list some of the best minerals and beneficial antioxidants found in foods and supplements to add to your arsenal to fight inflammation. This list is arranged in alphabetical order to make it easier to use as a reference tool.

BLUEBERRIES

Blueberries make the list as an antioxidant superfood. This dark, delicious fruit may be small, but it's crammed with antioxidants and phytoflavinoids. These tiny berries are high in potassium and vitamin C and work as an anti-inflammatory to aid in lowering the risk of heart disease and cancer. Strawberries, raspberries, and blackberries also contain anthocyanins, which provide anti-inflammatory effects.

AVOCADO

Avocados are packed with potassium, magnesium, and fiber. This savory fruit is another superfood rich in antioxidants and anti-inflammatory properties. They provide a great source of healthy unsaturated fat and are packed with potassium, magnesium, and fiber.

COENZYME Q10

Coenzyme Q10, also known as CoQ10, is another antioxidant that has been shown to have anti-inflammatory properties. It is found naturally in avocados, olive oil, parsley, peanuts, beef liver, salmon, sardines, mackerel, spinach, and walnuts.

GINGER

Ginger is comparative to the fact that it contains powerful anti-inflammatory compounds known as gingerols. Ginger root is found in the produce section at your grocery store and is available as a potent antioxidant supplement that helps prevent the oxidation of a damaging free radical called peroxynitrite. Ginger adds flavor to your favorite stir-fry, can be made into ginger tea, or can be taken as a supplement.

GLUTATHIONE

Glutathione is another antioxidant that fights free-radicals with anti-inflammatory properties. This is available as a supplement and is also available naturally in plant foods, including apples, asparagus, avocados, garlic, grapefruit, spinach, tomatoes, and milk thistle.

MAGNESIUM

Magnesium is a mineral supplement that can help reduce inflammation for those with low magnesium, which is linked to stress. Statistics suggest an estimated 70% of Americans are deficient in this mineral, which is surprising since it is readily available in a number of foods, including dark leafy greens, almonds, avocado, and many legumes.

SALMON

Salmon is rich in anti-inflammatory omega-3s. It is better to eat wild caught than farmed. It is best to try to include oily fish in your diet two times a week, and if you're not a fan of fish, then try a high-quality fish oil supplement.

VITAMIN B

People with low levels of vitamin B6 have a tendency to have high levels of C-reactive protein, which, as was mentioned in chapter 2, is a measure of inflammation in the body. B vitamins, including B6, can be found in vegetables like broccoli, bell peppers, cauliflower, kale, and mushrooms. It is also available in meats, including chicken, cod, turkey, and tuna.

Folate (B-9 in natural form) and folic acid (a synthetic form of B-9) is another B vitamin linked to the reduction of inflammation. A brief Italian study submits that even daily, short-term low dosages of folic acid supplements can lessen inflammation in overweight people. Folate is found in foods like asparagus, black-eyed peas, dark leafy greens, and lima beans.

VITAMIN D

Estimates suggest two-thirds of the people living in the U.S. are deficient in vitamin D. It's another vitamin that helps reduce inflammation, and getting insufficient amounts is linked to a range of inflammatory conditions. This vitamin is unique in that we get it naturally when we spend time in the sunshine with the important spectrum is ultraviolet B (UVB). It is also available as a supplement and is available in foods like egg yolks, fish, and organ meats, as well as foods that are supplemented with it. When choosing a Vitamin D supplement, look for Vitamin D3, which is the most bioavailable form of the vitamin. The ideal amount for supplementation is 5000IU per day, and many of these pills cost less than $7 for a 3 month supply.

VITAMIN E

Another potent antioxidant, this vitamin can aid in lessening inflammation. It is available as a quality supplement or can be found naturally in nuts and seeds and vegetables like avocado and spinach.

VITAMIN K

There are two kinds of vitamin K: K1 and K2. K1 is found in leafy greens, cabbage, and cauliflower. K2 is available in eggs and liver. This vitamin helps reduce inflammatory markers and may help to fight osteoporosis and heart disease.

CHAPTER 4: FOODS THAT REDUCE METABOLIC INFLAMMATION

Becoming healthier and more fit should be a primary goal that anyone should follow. Autophagy can help you achieve this goal, as it's responsible for destroying and recycling old and damaged cell parts, in order for your body to work better. It is usually linked with the fat burning process, as autophagy happens when the body runs on fat. It basically actions on the fat cells, in order to get the energy required for your brain and body. Ketosis and fasting can be intertwined, as ketosis is regarded as the first phase of Intermittent Fasting, during which ketones levels are higher. Ketosis is not the same thing as the keto-adaption process.

The first term describes a metabolic state with appropriate levels of ketones and blood sugar. During this phase, the insulin level and blood sugar decreases, whilst the ketones levels are increasing. This is generated by glucose deprivation, meaning that it took quite a while since the body last had its glucose required for energy. This substance can be found in all the carbs (and proteins as well) and is the primary source of energy for the body under "normal circumstances."

Speaking of glucose intake, the modern-day diet relies heavily on carbs because we mainly consume processed food. This means that the body mainly uses the glucose from the carbs, but the big problem is that it simply can't burn all the glycogen it gets, mainly because of the high carb intake, but also because of the passive lifestyle. Nowadays, around 70% of the diseases known to humans are caused by the food we eat, and high amounts of carbs can be blamed for this situation. In urban communities, where most people live, it's a little difficult to find natural and organic food, as everywhere you are bombarded by processed food. The sad truth is that most of the food we eat today is processed, and this comes with very high levels of carbs. What's even worse is that these types of food have little to nothing nutritional value and causes addiction. In order to cover your daily nutritional needs, you have to eat more, but this means a caloric boom.

Processed food is more caloric dense than nutrient dense, and this is a major disadvantage. When people are facing increased risks of chronic diseases like type 2 diabetes, heart, stomach, liver, and kidney diseases, it's clear that something has to be done to change the way we eat and also what we eat. Studies indicate that in order to become healthier and also thinner, you would need to decrease the glucose level when eating. This can happen by cutting down on carbs and, in some cases, also means protein limiting. When not burned, glucose gets stored is your blood, increasing the insulin and blood sugar level. Carbs consumption is like a vicious circle, as you easily get hungry after consuming food rich in carbs, and you are craving for more. But these meals come with strings attached, as you will get higher glucose levels and eventually higher blood sugar and insulin level. In order to make a radical change, you will need to make your body burn fat, not glucose. As you probably already have blood sugar, you will need to stop eating so many carbs, and therefore you will have less glucose to worry about. You can achieve this through fasting (restraining yourself from food) or through a special diet.

Traditional fasting means not consuming any food at all; some would not consume anything at all, just like religious fanatics during a special period, the Ramadan in the Islamic religion can be a perfect example. By not consuming anything at all, you are allowing your body to use the available glucose to be burnt, and once it has burned it all, the body will have to switch the energy source from glucose to fat. As the glucose level is decreasing, the same happens with the insulin level, setting it free to do its job and regulate the blood sugar.

The body easily adapts to such changes, and since its glucose reserves are running out, it has to figure out a way to use a different fuel type. That's where ketones step in, which is the necessary tool to break down fat cells and release the energy from them. You need to easily make the difference between ketosis and the keto-adapted process, as ketosis represents the metabolic state during which the ketone bodies are multiplying. The keto-adapted process is responsible for switching the energy source from glucose to fat. You can be in a ketosis state but still not running on fats and ketones for fuel.

Intermittent Fasting is more of a self-discipline process because it's about planning when to eat than what to eat. Limiting the feeding window to a limited amount of hours can give time for the body to process the food and use it for energy. However, when the body has already processed the food it has consumed, and it's not receiving anything else, it will start to look for a different alternative as fuel. The fat tissue is the most "to hand" option, and ketones can help extract the energy from it. If daily fasting has feeding and a fasting window, these terms are not the same with the fed and fasted state. The fed state represents the period of time required by your body to process the food it consumed, whilst the fasted state refers to the period after the fed state, during which the body doesn't have to process any food, and it's also not receiving any nutrients at all.

The fasted state starts approximately 12 hours after the last meal, and, coincidence or not, that's when ketosis starts. In the fasted state, the ketones levels are increasing rapidly, whilst the blood sugar and insulin levels are decreasing. At this point, the body doesn't have available glucose to burn, and it's looking for alternative fuel. Also, this is the right moment to apply stress to your body, and by stress, you need to understand the physical exercise. This will force the fat burning process, will increase even more the ketones levels, and the insulin will take care of the stored glucose from your blood.

CHAPTER 5: INTERMITTENT FASTING AND AUTOPHAGY

The concept of intermittent fasting means that you have to fast at regular intervals of the daily routine. The autophagy works tremendously under such circumstances, and with the passage of time, the working length can be achieved mordaciously. However, there are certain techniques that need to be compensated for while you are doing intermittent fasting. They are as follows:

1. THE KETOSIS STATES

It is a state of intermittent fasting in which the body is able to lower down its metabolic rate, and all the saturated fats located in various parts of the body are easily eliminated. You tend to start this while you are at the 12th hour of your body level, and this state forces you to be away from all those bad things that are quite hectic for your body. You become all composed and compassionate in yourself while you are on this diet, and thus, you are all good to come and proceed in the coming.

2. THE RECYCLING OF CELLS

During the second state of the body, the body is able to do the recycling of cells. The cell line is so lenient and efficient in this scenario that you become very effective in this regard. The recycling of cells is an autophagy process and helps to improve the circulation of blood in your holistically. Therefore, the use of autophagy is tremendously very effective for your body to work on, and with this, you are able to make a better transition in your body by all means necessary.

3. THE 54 HOURS SHIFT

By this state, the insulin level has dropped by 54 percent, and you are feeling very relaxed and better in your style. This the hours' shift that helps you to lessen any composed fat on your waistline, and with the passage of time, you are able to be very strong and sustainable in your requirement. Therefore, these three stages are a must to learn states of intermittent fasting, and anyone who desires to have an autophagy run in it, the 54 hours shift is the best shift for it.

INCORPORATING INTERMITTENT FASTING

In order to incorporate intermittent fasting in you. You have to adopt the following things in yourself.

1. BE PATIENT AND COMPOSED

This means that any diet that has a good number of intakes in it and can deliver a better potential in you with the passage of time, is essential and effective for you. The idea in this scenario is that you have to look for diet and body ideas that can be helpful for you on a coherent level and could engage the best out of you. This might be a little problematic at first, but with the passage of time, you will be able to harness it.

2. ALWAYS LOOK FOR A GREEN DIET

The green diet will help you to pay a better benefit to your body. You will be able to see how the body language is able to incorporate better standings in you, and with the passage of time, you are able to furnish yourself to the next level. Therefore, it is important for you to understand that looking for a green diet for you is the best thing that ever happened to you, and you must incorporate it in the coming time.

INTO YOUR WORKOUT PLAN

The keto diet and the process of autophagy should be incorporated into your workout plan. You must be able to see how the workout is able to make you stand out in front of any issue. You must incorporate physical exercises that could be very effective for your brain and could make you very established in physique as well. Therefore, the incorporation of a workout plan is necessary for you to understand how the body is being moved with possible direction and how autophagy can help to relate in this manner.

CHAPTER 6: PRECAUTIONS TO TAKE REGARDING AUTOPHAGY AND FASTING

Fasting has a lot of advantages. However, fasting is not meant for everyone. To better understand the theory of fasting, let us compare Fasting to a tool (such as an arrow), which can either be used properly or misused. Holding to that, we will use the archery metaphor to explain the effective use and the misuse of fasting/autophagy. A hunter could have different sizes and tips of arrows in his quiver. When he finds an antelope, he will use a sharp wooden arrow, but when he faces a lion or bear, he would go for something stronger: probably an arrow with metallic tips. The point is not to use the wrong method for the right purpose.

WHO SHOULD AVOID FASTING

Pregnant and breastfeeding mothers. Whether you have a child you're breastfeeding or one who is still in your uterus, you need all the calories you can get; both the mother and the infant need to be fed well to stay nourished and healthy.

Underaged students and those below 18 should avoid Fasting. Children under the age of 18 are still growing and need all the vital nutrients and minerals to have healthy growth and development.

Those that are underweight and/or malnourished. If you find it difficult to tell whether you are malnourished or not, you could ask your physician or a trusted friend. Those having an eating disorder such as bulimia are included in this category.

Individuals who have Type-2 Diabetes. Fasting has been used over the years as a means of reversing the effect of Type-2 diabetes. However, you still need to consult your physician before beginning a fast.

WHO NEEDS TO BE CAUTIOUS?

Another group of individuals who also need to be cautious is those with occasional gastroesophageal reflux disease (GERD). Those who fall into this category need to check with their physician as well if they wish to fast and must be closely monitored.

There are solid pieces of evidence to prove that GERD could be aggravated by fasting and the symptoms could become worsened. This possible worsening is because during fasting, the stomach will be devoid of food, and there will be nothing which the gastric juice would digest.

Individuals on medications need to be cautious while fasting as the fasting periods could overlap when such drugs would be taken, especially those medications that would require you to eat before using them.

In addition, those on cancer therapy and other medical treatment must be cautious and should have an in-depth discussion with their physician before fasting.

CHAPTER 7: INTERMITTENT WATER FASTING

Water is life. No cell in your body can function without it. No living thing on Earth can exist without water's vital essence. Because performance autophagy relates to cell tissue cleansing and renewal, without water, this process would be null and void. The basic human cell is protein, fat, cholesterol, and water. While you begin to increase autophagy through fasting and ketosis, you begin the process of reducing wastes and toxins in the body on a cellular level.

Water will get used to performing all these functions, collecting and disposing of the exhausted materials and compounds. The point of energy is to give life to our experience. The point of water is to give life to that energy. Because water is so significant to the system as a whole, water fasting is a described method of autophagy on account of its ability to enhance autophagic reaction and response.

Timing is everything. Intermittence is a level of time that allows your body to receive ample energy through healthy eating and diet, followed by moments and periods of fasting. This alternating effect brings about effective autophagy, giving space and time to the cells to renew and for the body to gain nutrients; both are necessary for optimal health.

Water fasting is the method by which all food is eliminated slowly over the course of several hours and/or days to allow your body time to gently respond and react to fewer calories. Water is then increased to allow for proper autophagic response and activity. The only thing consumed in water fast is water; however, some vitamins and minerals may be consumed for proper internal balance. Although no calories are ingested, some vitamins and minerals are necessary for the proper function of the cells so that they may do their work during autophagy.

Water is essential; it carries all life and acts as the conduit of all internal function and performance. Without it, autophagy wouldn't work. Balancing the fast with extra water is key to healthy autophagic response and brings about greater change, renewal, and deep cellular healing.

CHAPTER 8: COMMON KINDS OF WATER FASTING

There are many different ways that you can perform a water fast. All these types of fasting will offer you benefits; it's up to you to select one that suits your individual needs, your lifestyle requirements, and your end goal.

1. DRY FASTING

This fast is the most extreme and often called the *Absolute Fast*. The roots of dry fasting are spiritual and consists of foregoing water and food for short periods. We do not necessarily recommend this, as it is really only for very experienced fasters.

2. LIQUID FASTING

This is fasting using only liquids – no food is consumed whatsoever. This can be any liquid or can be more specific as shown by the types of fast that follow.

3. JUICE FASTING

This fast includes some nutritional value just in a pure, or natural, form and is very popular. This is because almost any vegetable, fruit, or juice can be blended with the powerful juicers that are currently on the market.

4. WATER FASTING

This fast may be the oldest of its kind and is thought to provide the greatest physically therapeutic benefit in a shorter period of time, because the detoxification process happens quickly. Water fasting is also the easiest type of liquid fasting.

5. MASTER CLEANSE

This is a relatively new method, which is often called the *Lemonade Diet.*

Master Cleanse Recipe

Combine:

- 8 oz purified water

- 2 tbl lime or lemon juice, fresh squeezed

- 2 tbl maple syrup, 100% pure

- a dash cayenne pepper

Recipe yields one 10 oz serving. Drink the mixture anytime through the day, up to 12 glasses daily.

Here are *some tips if you decide that this is the diet for you*:

- If you are prone to hypoglycemia, Master Cleanse is not recommended due to its high sugar levels.

- The night before you plan to start this fast, drink one cup of herbal laxative tea.

- Blend up enough for each day's serving before your first meal, adding the pepper and lemon fresh as you pour each drink, and plan on consuming 6-12 glasses per day.

- Plan on using lemons at room temperature. To best release the juices, roll them, applying firm pressure, back and forth across the countertop right before juicing.

- Don't worry about feeling lightheaded or dizzy. You could be consuming about 650-1300 calories per day from the syrup.

- Drink one cup of herbal laxative tea every evening during your fast.

- After using the Master Cleanse for 10 days, take 3 days for a successful transition back to solid foods. On Day 1, drink several glasses of orange juice throughout the day. On Day 2, eat fresh fruit and drink orange juice and vegetable broth. On Day 3, include fresh vegetables with Day 2's list of food and drinks. Return to a normal diet on the following day.

6. SELECTIVE FASTING

Selective fasting, sometimes known as *partial fasting*, combines liquid fasting with some solid food. It could range from a little bit to a lot based on your needs. You can even choose to combine some of these fasting techniques to fit around you!

CHAPTER 9: WEIGHTLOSS AND WATER FASTING

There have been a number of different kinds of weight loss programs you may have come across in recent times. From choosing weight loss supplements to enrolling for exercise regimes that may seem completely out of place to adapting to a diet that you may believe works well in your favor, weight loss is something you can't get out of your mind when you are overweight. However, when it comes to losing weight, you need to keep in mind that it's not a temporary solution that you should rely on. Relying on these will help you get to the desired weight before you decide to go back to your old habits.

Weight loss is all about changing the way you look at life and incorporating certain techniques that will benefit you in the long run and keep you healthy from within as well. A common misconception with weight is that if you are not overweight, you are healthy. The truth, however, is people who aren't that heavy may also suffer from a number of health conditions because of damaged cells in their body, and this is why you need to consider leading a healthy lifestyle rather than obsessing over weight loss or weight management. Having said that, adapting to autophagy has a number of benefits, and weight loss is definitely one of them. The only difference between the weight loss program that autophagy has to offer versus other weight loss programs is that autophagy benefits you from within.

LOSING WEIGHT FOR THE LOOKS

The most obvious reason somebody wants to lose weight is to look good.

When you are a few pounds overweight, your confidence level automatically starts to drop, and a feeling of inferiority starts to seep in. While you should always be confident about the way you look, if you are not happy with your appearance, you should do something to change it.

There are tons of people who start getting depressed because of their weight, mainly because they can't manage to get in shape no matter what they do. The main reason you might not be able to lose weight is because of low metabolism levels. If your metabolism rate is low, no matter how much you diet or starve yourself, you are not going to get in shape. It is important for you to adapt to autophagy so that you start off the process of weight loss and you boost your metabolism rate in order for your body to start burning fat. This is not going to happen overnight, which is why you have to prepare yourself for long-term results. Do not look for shortcuts.

The problem with most weight loss programs today is that they promote weight loss as a trophy for something that you will do for the next thirty days. Simply popping a pill or following a diet plan only for a month to lose weight is the worst thing you can do to yourself. Not only will this affect your body internally, but it will also reflect on your appearance. While some of these weight loss solutions help you to get in shape, they end up giving you horrible skin, tired eyes, and severe hair loss. This is caused because of the lack of nutrients in your system.

If you want to get healthy and you want to do it the right way, you have to give your body time. Autophagy isn't as popular as other quick weight loss solutions because it's not a quick fix. It is a longtime commitment that you have to make, not only so that you look great but also so that you feel amazing from within and you wave goodbye to illnesses.

LOSING WEIGHT TO GET HEALTHY

As mentioned earlier, most weight loss solutions are so that you look great physically, but what you really need is one that makes you healthy from within. One of the most important things you need to understand is that losing weight isn't just about looking great, but also getting healthy at the same time. In order for you to do that, you have to choose something that benefits your body internally as well as externally. The reason autophagy is so great is that it helps with repairing your body from within, and you will also be able to see the results externally.

The main difference between a short-term weight loss program and the autophagy way of life lies in the name itself. A short-term weight loss solution will give you short-term results, and you will eventually end up gaining weight and suffer from a number of health problems. Once you activate autophagy, not only will you start losing weight, but you'll get healthy, and this is essential in order for you to keep illnesses away.

Autophagy helps you to reverse the signs of aging because it repairs the cells in your body, and this keeps a number of age-related diseases away, making it a long-term and effective solution that grows on you. While it's not the easiest weight loss process to get used to, it is something that you will learn to adapt and manage to incorporate for the rest of your life so that you lead a healthy life and focus on being healthy rather than just looking great.

CHAPTER 10: INTERMITTENT FASTING COULD HELP YOU AGE SLOWLY

One of the biggest benefits of autophagy is seen in the anti-aging effect, which arises when you restrict calorie intake, this makes autophagy possible.

One of the major characteristics of a young organism is a high rate of autophagy. With time, however, autophagy reduces and sets the stage for cell damage. By seeking ways to induce autophagy via fasting, you can slow down aging. We age when there are lots of damaged cells, as well as an inability to recycle old cells.

From the above, it is evident that aging and autophagy seem to be linked. Without enough autophagy in mammals, degeneration of cells follows. This degeneration manifests as aging, which is linked to reduced autophagy. This is why autophagy is an effective tool to mitigate aging.

To understand the relationship between autophagy and aging, a knowledge of how cells replicate is vital. The human body has more than 100 trillion cells (Atkinson, 2018), of which more than 200 billion cells undergo division daily. At times, these cells get sick and worn out, so when they divide, they will produce more sick and weak cells. With time, the higher the number of sick and damaged body cells, the more you age. This is where autophagy comes in, as a means to repair these damaged cells to make them young and healthy again.

We have established autophagy as the internal cellular repair process. In simple terms, autophagy targets old and weak cells, refurbishes them to make them healthy while getting rid of others.

AUTOPHAGY LOWERS RISK OF NEURODEGENERATIVE DISEASE

With time, a man grows; he gets subjected to the disease of the aging brain. However, these ailments might take a while to manifest because of the presence of proteins in the brain cells, protein cells that are not acting right. Autophagy will get rid of this protein, reducing its tendency to accumulate.

For Alzheimer's disease, for instance, autophagy helps get rid of amyloid while it gets rid of α-synuclein in Parkinson's disease. One of the reasons dementia is thought to be related to diabetes is because excessive high blood sugar suppresses autophagy. These make it difficult to cleanse the cells.

AUTOPHAGY IMPROVES SKIN HEALTH

The skin is the largest organ in the body. This makes it susceptible to damage from elements like weather changes, chemicals, light, heat, humidity, and other physical damage. The skin takes a lot from the environment, and it is a miracle that it does not look horrible due to wear and tear. The skin, however, with time, undergoes a lot of damage and toxins, which triggers aging.

Although the body is constantly making new cells, with autophagy you can repair the existing ones, which results in glowing, youthful skin. It is also important to note that skin cells engulf bacteria that are harmful to the body. This explains why it is important to have autophagy as a care mechanism for the skin.

CHAPTER 11: HOW TO FAST CORRECTLY

Before you think about fasting, you need to know your limits. Fasting isn't something that you just jump headfirst into without any preparation or research. Your experience, health condition, daily nutrition, and the relationship you have with food need to be evaluated before you decide to start fasting.

EXPERIENCE AND DURATION

If you are not experienced at fasting, then I recommend that you don't start with a 21-day water fast on your first attempt. You may also have found some information online that might have painted a rather rosy picture about all the benefits that you can reap by going on an extreme diet like a dry fast.

A juice cleanse is a partial fast, and it gives your body some time to get used to the idea of fasting, so I recommend that you start with a simple form of fasting before you opt for a stringent one. Also, ensure that you are aware of all the possible side effects of a fast before you start one. Start with an easy form of intermittent fasting and make your way up to an alternate day fasting plan.

One of the reasons why you must ease into fasting is to understand the way in which your body responds to fasting. If you know what you can expect, then you are in a better position to deal with issues when they come up. Being prepared for expected challenges makes it easier to fast.

HEALTH

Forget about the saying, "feed a cold, starve a fever." You need to focus on your general health and not just your immediate weight loss goals before you start fasting. If you are fasting as a means to detox your body from a junk food binge, then come up with an alternative or healthy diet plan before fasting.

You must remember that your overall health is more important than anything else that might come your way. If you are on the list of people I mentioned above, then refrain from fasting at all costs. If you don't pay attention to your health, it will land you in a lot of trouble, so please consult your doctor before you start fasting or making any changes to your diet.

NUTRITION AND HYDRATION

Are you wondering what nutrition I am talking about while fasting? You need to understand that your body has a natural inbuilt reserve of certain key nutrients, like fat-soluble vitamins, that help with regular functioning of the cells when you aren't eating.

You need to ensure that your body has plenty of water-soluble minerals and vitamins while fasting. This means that you need to ensure that your body has sufficient electrolytes within it to function normally. If your body starts running out of these important electrolytes, it will lead to dehydration and will have a negative effect on your body's metabolism.

An essential form of nourishment that your body needs is water. It is not only necessary for transporting nutrients in the body, but it is also important for water removal and the regulation of your body temperature. Water provides a medium within which all other metabolic processes take place, so you need to ensure that your body is thoroughly hydrated at all times.

A lot of fasters tend to experience dehydration because their bodies aren't getting the usual volume of food, and it means that they will need to make up for this deficit. The best way to do this and eliminate any of the negative effects of dehydration is to keep your body thoroughly hydrated.

RELATIONSHIP WITH FOOD

All those who are experiencing any eating disorders or have suffered from any in the past need to avoid fasting until they have overcome those issues. It might seem quite appealing to fast, but it can lead to a relapse of any unhealthy condition.

If you have any history of food abuse or you use food to cope with emotional stress or trauma, then the first thing that you must do is work on developing a healthy relationship with food before you think about fasting. If you don't, then it will only lead to additional stress that is rather unnecessary.

You will learn more about the different tips that you can follow while you are fasting in the coming chapters. Each person has a different response to intermittent fasting. You will never be able to gauge how your body will react to fasting by comparing yourself to the people around you.

You will need to see how your body reacts and make any changes required. What might work for one person might not work for you, and that's perfectly all right. Everyone is different, so the best thing that you can do is to listen to your body. Your body knows what it wants, so learn to listen to it. Also, while you are fasting, you need to take it easy on your exercise regime for a couple of days. Give your body and yourself some time to get used to your new diet.

CHAPTER 12: AUTOPHAGY, KETOSIS, AND FASTING

Autophagy is an important process that restores worn-out cells during starvation and fasting. It is a critical aspect of anti-aging and longevity experienced in caloric restriction. Fasting is one of the most effective methods of increasing autophagy.

Ketosis refers to the metabolic state of high ketone utilization and production. It occurs when your body's glycogen stores are suppressed, and the liver generates ketones that replace glucose. You can experience ketosis during fasting or when under a low carb ketogenic diet.

Ketosis and autophagy support each other even though they are not mutually inclusive. Still, you can be in ketosis without autophagy, and you can experience autophagy without ketosis. It is only that you will see them together because they share similar principles.

DOES AUTOPHAGY NEED KETOSIS

Here's what controls autophagy and ketosis:

- **Autophagy is stimulated under energy deprivation caused by a deficiency of amino acid, fasting, thermoregulation, and glucose restriction. In metabolism, you will require little insulin, high AMPK, and low Mtor.**

- **Ketosis is attained when there is glucose restriction. The main feature that leads to the development of ketone bodies is carbohydrate deficiencies and glycogen depletion. Protein can also lead to carbohydrate synthesis via gluconeogenesis.**

However, it is secondary and doesn't impact ketosis that much. As a result, you don't need low insulin or low Mtor, although it always happens.

You can experience ketosis while consuming high amounts of Mtor and higher insulin because you consumed something that contains high levels of protein. It will regulate nutritional ketosis and high level of ketones, but it will inhibit autophagy because of the high nutrient content aspect of Mtor that prevents autophagy.

Autophagy doesn't need ketosis to be stimulated because you can fast for up to 3 days and still not experience ketosis, based on the nature of your keto-adaptation. But remaining in ketosis fulfills most of the prerequisite of autophagy-like low blood glucose, low insulin, and lower Mtor. You only need to base it on the period you have been fasting for.

MEASURE KETONES TO DETERMINE AUTOPHAGY

There are no genuine methods to measure autophagy in human beings, but it can be estimated by reviewing the glucose ketone index and the ratio of insulin to glucagon.

Lower insulin to glucagon ratio indicates more ketogenesis, fat oxidation, catabolism, and nutrient deprivation.

A higher ratio of insulin to glucagon indicates more anabolism, increased blood sugar, higher insulin, and nutrient storage.

The glucose ketone index reveals an estimated ratio of insulin-glucagon with a lower score reflecting higher ketosis and more AMPK.

The time it takes before autophagy starts depends on the nutrient status of your body and the availability of specific nutrients, especially glucose and ketones.

If you are not eating a lot of carbs or too much protein daily, then you can expect autophagy to kick in faster than that person who has to burn through those calories first.

AUTOPHAGY ON KETO

Experiencing ketosis while consuming the ketogenic diet can boost the autophagy process and recycle unique proteins via chaperone-mediated autophagy. This can still happen even while eating as long as your carbs and protein remain low.

A ketogenic diet can limit neuronal injury through autophagy and mitochondrial pathways in seizures. It emulates a lot of features of the fasted physiology like Mtor and lowers insulin.

However, the ketogenic diet emulates most of the benefits of fasting and probably helps stimulate autophagy faster than other diets. But for that to succeed, you would require to adhere to the real therapeutic macros of 5% carbs, 70-80% fat, and 15-20% protein. Many people eat a lot of protein and carbs, which is better but it's not going to regulate a constant state of autophagy.

Consuming a low carb ketogenic diet that regulates carbs and doesn't over-do protein is a great basal template for controlling good metabolic health and being ready to get into autophagy faster.

Besides fasting, the therapeutic ketogenic diet that includes some type of intermittent fasting and not more than 2 meals per day is the nearest thing you can get to an autophagy-mimicking diet.

Eating once every day on a keto combined with exercise, consuming autophagic foods, and exposure to other hermetic stressors is one of the most autophagy boosts you can attain while sticking within the 24-hour period. In general, the actual benefits of autophagy start after 24 hours and extend for 3-5 days of fasting.

ARE KETONES THE BEST FUEL FOR BURNING FAT?

If you have ever been to a gas station to pump fuel into your car, you must have seen these three numbers (87-89-93) listed on the pump. But what do they really represent? Maybe someone has ever told you that those numbers represent the rating of something known as octane, which defines the level of compression a fuel can endure before igniting. The higher octane means, the less likely the fuel is going to pre-ignite at higher pressures and destroy your engine.

Your body is like a car because it needs fuel to run. Food is your octane, but you can choose the type of fuel to use. You can decide to run on a low octane(sugar) or a high octane(fat). Feeding your body with sugar fuel is likely to cause your body to burst out with fat and be destroyed with chronic disease. On the flip side, fat fuel is highly efficient and will ensure you remain lean.

HOW KETONES ARE GENERATED

Ketones are generated when very little amounts of carbs are consumed, and the body breaks down fats. As a result, it produces fatty acids, which are burned off within the liver through beta-oxidation. Similar to fats, carbs are one of the major food types. But carbs change into sugar when synthesized by the body, which results in obesity and health challenges. Alternatively, the human brain and body prefer ketones as its main energy source because it runs 70 percent more efficiently than sugar.

From an evolutionary perspective, this preference looks sensible. Keeping in mind that carbs were not easily accessible during prehistoric days.

WHY YOU NEED TO MAKE KETONES YOUR MAIN FUEL

The state in which the body processes ketones as its major fuel is known as ketosis. Ketones are produced when the body has an insufficient amount of sugar. When the body is deficient in sugar, you switch to ketosis.

Your body needs the energy to control metabolism. This energy is kept as glycogen or fat. Until your body requires energy, glycogen is stored inside the skeletal muscles and liver. When glycogen is stored in your body, it is changed into sugar when needed. Because it is easier for your body to utilize this energy, you have to use it before it starts to burn fat. In the absence of glycogen, your body will convert stored fat into ketones.

A typical human being has around 600 grams of glycogen inside the body. This is approximately 500 grams in skeletal muscles and 100 grams in the liver.

WHAT FOODS TO EAT TO PRODUCE KETONES

Diet experts have marketed the keto diet because it is effective at burning fat. However, most keto diet resources don't talk about the right foods and nutrients that stimulate cravings. As a result, humans continue to gain weight and grow unhealthy bodies. That is why you need to carefully consider the foods you eat while using ketones to decrease body fat.

It is good to take seafood, pasture-raised eggs, and grass-fed meats because they add protein to your body. Take in carbohydrates from dark green leafy vegetables, and it should make around 5-10% of your diet.

Don't forget to include berries. They are best for low sugar content and high levels of phytonutrients, so you should include blackberries, blueberries, and raspberries. Include a serving of berries daily for its excellent antioxidant protection.

IS IT POSSIBLE TO INDUCE AUTOPHAGY WITHOUT STARVING YOURSELF?

While fasting is the easiest route to turn off nutrient-sensing pathways, but that is not for everyone, as we shall see later. Despite that, most of the physiological responses of a ketogenic diet emulate fasting, and the drop in insulin that happens along with the diet is in part responsible.

If conducted well, the ketogenic diet will trigger the metabolic condition of ketosis where blood ketones have been increased. Beta-hydroxybutyrate, the main ketone body, has been found to activate chaperone-mediated autophagy in vitro. But this was in the context of nutrient deprivation.

CHAPTER 13: HYPERTROPHIC GROWTH

Those that train for strength and sports performance have consistently criticized those who partake in bodybuilding training. Often claiming training for aesthetics is inefficient because optimizing strength, speed, and athleticism should be the primary objective. While there is some truth to this, having more muscle tissue is crucial for many sports and for general health. The key is to train for hypertrophy without sacrificing mobility, speed, body composition, or overall fitness.

Although hypertrophy training is not the most efficient way to build strength, it still offers many benefits to sports performance:

- If two muscles have the same cross-sectional area of muscle fibers, the one with bigger fibers will be stronger.

- Increased GPP (General Physical Preparedness). Hypertrophy training increases work capacity and will allow an athlete to recover faster over time.

- Increased glycogen storage.

- Increased fat oxidation.

- Mass moves Mass. In many sports, having more body weight offers a large benefit, but it is important to make sure this weight is functional muscle instead of body fat.

Studies consistently show that compound barbell exercises are the best when trying to stimulate an anabolic hormone response and increase muscle mass. This is why the primary movements in this program will be the squat, bench, deadlift, and overhead press. There will also be assistance exercises that will all be completed with a barbell as well. The goal with these movements is to focus on moving the maximum load possible while remaining proper technique. On top of building muscle, a byproduct of this program will be an increase in strength. I personally compete in powerlifting and have set personal records coming right out of this program.

I have implemented several key principles to the PERFORMANCE HYPERTROPHY PROGRAM:

- *Submaximal Loads:* All prescribed training loads in this program will remain under 90% of the 1RM (1 rep max). Many studies show how beneficial the minimum effective dose really is. You can stimulate close to the same effect with a lesser load but also recover much quicker and not inhibit performance on the following training days. Lifting with a maximal load, like in a traditional powerlifting program, does not allow for the amount of training volume this program requires. Also, the risk of injury is greatly decreased when training with weights that are easily lifted.

- *Undulating Periodization:* Undulating periodization adjusts the volume and intensity of each lift within each week. If the program calls for a heavy squat this week, deadlifts will be lighter. This will allow the lifter to lift heavier and recover quicker. Linear periodization, which has been widely used by many for years, is dead. It's outdated and definitely not applicable to high-level athletes.

- *No Weak Links:* The assistance exercises in the program will be variations attacking weaknesses in the athlete's physique. In any athletic scenario, the individual can only perform as well as their weakest link. By attacking these head on, we will correct dysfunction, increase performance, and decrease the risk of injury.

- *Recover, Recover, Recover:* There are only four workout days per week in this program, and that is very important. When focusing on hypertrophy, the recovery periods are more important than lifting. On these recovery days, take the opportunity to focus on mobility and overall health. Lower intensity yoga is highly suggested.

- *Caloric Surplus:* When trying to build muscle, a caloric surplus is essential. A pound of muscle requires an additional 2,500 calories, so make sure to eat enough food. Focus on protein as much as possible.

It must be understood that this program is for intermediate to advanced lifters only. These barbell movements come with a higher risk of injury, so if you are not proficient in these exercises, please seek the help of a fitness professional or look to one of our beginner programs.

CHAPTER 14: LONGEVITY AND AUTOPHAGY

Taking care of your health doesn't have to make you feel like you're doing a chore or restricting yourself. Even if you're not keen on fasting, or if you simply want to opt out of a restrictive diet and eat normally, there are ways to guarantee that you activate autophagy to improve your well-being.

The key is to balance your diet according to your daily needs, and for that, you must choose your foods wisely. In each food category, there are substances that can prevent aging and trigger autophagy. While there aren't specific substances in food that are known to target autophagic regulation, you can fill your plate with a few options that will surely boost the benefits of existing autophagic processes.

Antioxidant-rich foods are an example. Mainly found in vegetables, antioxidants are molecules that function as a defense against free radicals. They can be produced by the body, but diet is a great source and can also stimulate the body to produce a greater amount of these protectors of the body.

It's as simple as following a color code: the more colorful, the more antioxidant-rich foods are. Red-colored foods, such as tomatoes, contain the substance lycopene. It helps to remove a part of the oxygen we breathe called free radicals. They are linked to degenerative processes like cancer and aging of the body. Fruits still have great antioxidant power, as they protect the body from the harmful action of free radicals. Lycopene has an important anti-aging function in protecting the prostate and cardiovascular system. The substance is always better absorbed by the body along with extra virgin olive oil, which helps in lowering bad cholesterol.

Soy has high levels of isoflavones, vitamins, fibers, and minerals, therefore, it has a multitude of benefits: reduces the risk of breast cancer, helps menopausal symptoms, and contains effective coadjuvants to prevent prostate cancer and osteoporosis. Yogurt is also another great friend of longevity. It is rich in calcium. The yogurt also has bacteria, the family lactobacillus, which are beneficial to the body, as well as being able to protect the intestinal tract against infections. (*Lv, X., Liu, S. and Hu, Z. 2017*)

Vegetables, broccoli, and cauliflower have nutrients such as the compound sulforaphane, which can destroy carcinogenic substances. Spinach and orange, on the other hand, contain iron and folic acid, which prevents the irritation of blood vessels and consequently heart attacks. It also contains two nutrients that lower your chances of developing blindness. Chestnut and fish, such as salmon and sardines, have omega-3 fat. It lowers the level of bad cholesterol and triglycerides, types of fats that can be produced by the body or ingested through food. Fibers found in cereals, nuts, pumpkin seeds, and sesame seeds also help lower cholesterol. (*Law, B., Chan, W. et al. 2014*)

All these effects are synergistic with autophagy, so it is important to consume a variety of foods rich in antioxidants. Eating a diet rich in antioxidants has been shown to promote health and longevity. In fact, some types of antioxidants have been associated with a 30% reduction in mortality in older adults.

CHAPTER 15: OXIDATIVE STRESS AND YOUR HORMONES

Aging is a continuous and progressive physiological process, where there's a decline in biological functions, as previously seen. This decline during aging is directly associated with an increased chance of developing neurodegenerative diseases. If you depend on other people to complete simple tasks on a daily basis, for example, you may have a higher risk of developing memory problems or see your cognitive capacities reduced.

There are other psychosocial implications in aging that we are often not aware of and which are determinant in the life of the elderly. A decline in the quantity and quality of social life are inevitable as we age. This factor can exacerbate biological factors that contribute to decline and further aggravate health problems. Thus, we can conclude that aging is a multifactorial process, dependent on genetic factors and individual habits. Habits can increase the susceptibility to develop diseases, and the psychological implications appear as an interdependent factor in aggravating diseases such as neurological pathologies. (*Nixon, R., 2013; Komatsu, M. et al., 2006; Shacka, J., 2008*)

In addition to this gradual loss of the capacity to perform physiological functions and to trigger adaptive responses, there's an increase in functional and structural impairment of different systems, including the central nervous system. One of the hallmarks of aging in the nervous system is the natural formation of senile plaques. These plaques, composed of protein aggregates, were linked to natural cell death and cognitive function deterioration in neuropathologies such as Alzheimer's disease, Parkinson's, amyotrophic lateral sclerosis, among others. Sporadic forms of these diseases make up the majority of observed cases, and their pathological basis is similar. It's still unclear how these factors initiate the neurodegenerative process, as they are heavily interconnected. Studies in molecular biology of aging have identified key cellular changes that can aggravate the existent damage and lead to neuronal death. (*Shacka, J., 2008; Wong, E. and Cuervo, A., 2010; Ghavami, S. et al., 2014*)

Cellular dysfunction due to protein aggregation is related to the damage of the organelles and vesicles traffic in general. Neuronal survival depends on the integrity and functionality of mitochondria. Mitochondria produce energy for the cell and protect the cell from oxidative stress, functioning as a cell quality checkpoint. Cumulative stress as a person ages is involved in early neurodegeneration and undermines this quality control. Thus, the mitochondria become more vulnerable, and the damage caused increases the levels of reactive species, which in turn influence the mitochondria's capacity to produce energy. (*Ghavami, S. et al., 2014; Tsai, S. et al., 2014*)

With aging there is also an increase of ROS related toxicity in the central nervous system, preceding protein aggregation and neuronal loss, as ROS removal mechanisms also suffer damage. We can mention the superoxide dismutase (SOD) and catalase (CAT) systems, which remove superoxide anions and hydrogen peroxide from the cytoplasm. Decreases in metabolic waste removal rates are also linked with an imbalance of neuronal homeostasis.

Changes in protein quality control and apoptotic pathways are also observed. Intracellular degradation processes such as autophagy can be heavily influenced by this gradual change in cellular biodynamics, and vice-versa. Some proteins involved in this pathway play a central role in neurodegeneration. For example, the ULK-1/Beclin-1 complex, involved in the initial phases of autophagocytosis, generate vesicles with a double lipid layer. The equivalent of Beclin-1 in yeast autophagy models is atg6, which participates in yeast's cellular survival mechanisms. A dysfunction in atg6 was proved to induce cancer and neurodegeneration. (*Cai, Y., Arikkath, J., 2016; Ghavami, S. et al., 2014*)

Another important protein in this system is LC3II, which is often used as a marker of autophagy. It was originally identified as a microtubule-associated protein and associates with the autophagosome membrane. LC3I is cytosolic, and LC3II is associated with the autophagic membrane. The detection of LC3I and LC3II is a sensitive marker for distinguishing and studying autophagosomes and is useful for monitoring the state of autophagocytosis since the conversion between LC3I in LC3II correlates with the number of autophagosomes.

As aging progresses, increasing evidence indicates that there is a reduction in the rate of autophagosome formation, maturation, and the fusion of these with the lysosome. Deficiencies in intracellular degradation processes are associated with the formation of protein aggregates characteristic of various neurodegenerative diseases and aging. It has even been shown that cell degradation pathways are impaired in patients suffering from neurodegeneration. More recently, Heng et al. have described the early impairment of the autophagocytic system in Huntington's disease model mice and its possible implication for protein aggregation and cell injury.

Deficiency in autophagy, in particular, is associated with neurodegenerative diseases such as Alzheimer's, Huntington's, Parkinson's, and frontotemporal lobar dementia. The evidence is that the accumulation of autophagosomes in the degenerating brain is associated with the progression of neurological diseases, but the exact relation between the autophagic function of the cell and the appearance of neurodegenerative states still needs to be studied. (*Wong, E. and Cuervo, A., 2010; Komatsu, M., et al. 2006*)

Zheng et al. showed that lysosomal changes appear in the early stages of axonal degeneration, and the maintenance of the function of these organelles could be important in delaying the progression of neurodegenerative diseases. More recently, Ma et al. demonstrated that there is an increase in autophagic activity at the onset of aging in senescence mice. This autophagic activity then decreases with the advancement of age culminating with pathological cellular alterations similar to the characteristics of sporadic Alzheimer's disease.

Disorders in the processes of intracellular degradation may contribute to the deposition of proteins in the brain. In addition, there is evidence that the involvement of the autophagolysosome complex is related to the appearance of Alzheimer's disease characteristics in an experimental model of neurodegeneration. To illustrate the importance of maintaining this system, Cuervo et al. demonstrated that basal suppression of macroautophagy in the brain of mice resulted in protein accumulation and neurodegeneration. In addition, these same authors have demonstrated that α-synuclein can directly damage the lysosomal system.

CHAPTER 16: FINDING THE LONG-TERM AND SHORT-TERM BENEFITS OF AUTOPHAGY

Autophagy helps maintain homeostasis. What is homeostasis? Balanced cellular function in the body is known as homeostasis. Homeostasis, as well as vibrant health, is the result of the p62 protein working its magic during autophagy. As a result of this, all the damaged cells that are accumulated in the body over time are removed, and this creates space for new cells to form. This process does sound good, but how does autophagy benefit you? Here are the benefits of autophagy.

IT CAN BE LIFE-SAVING

It might sound a tad dramatic, but it is quite true. It is scientifically proven. Autophagy's main purpose is life preservation. During times of severe stress like infection or even starvation, this process is kick-started, and it helps optimize the process of repair while reducing damage.

Intermittent fasting activates autophagy and can starve any infectious intruder of glucose. This reduces inflammation so that it is easier for the immune system to take necessary action and help repair the damage that this inflammation and infection has caused. In short, the autophagy mechanism has evolved in such a manner that it helps save energy and repair damage when energy is scarce, but it is also important for the immune system's defense mechanism to fight any illness.

MAY PROMOTE LONGEVITY

Anti-aging benefits certainly sound mythical, almost like a unicorn.

Beauty isn't merely skin deep, and it runs deeper. Scientists discovered autophagy during the 50s, and since then there have been several studies that were and are still being conducted to understand the manner in which autophagy improves cellular function and health.

Instead of absorbing any new nutrients, during autophagy, cells tend to replace their damaged parts, get rid of any toxic material within, and start to fix themselves. When the cells in the body begin to repair themselves, they certainly tend to work better, and they act like younger cells.

You might have noticed some people have a different biological age and a different chronological age. The toxic damage that your body experiences and its ability to repair this situation plays a significant role in these differences.

BETTER METABOLISM

Autophagy is similar to a housekeeping service. Not only does it take the trash out, but also it replaces different vital cell parts like the mitochondria. Mitochondria are the powerhouse in a cell that not only burns fat and produces ATP, but is also your body's energy currency. Any buildup of toxins in the mitochondria doesn't just damage cells, and if these cells are destroyed proactively, it helps save future wear and tear of the cells.

Autophagy helps your cells function more effectively and efficiently, and it also helps synthesize new proteins. All this makes your cells quite healthy and this, in turn, improves your metabolism.

REDUCTION OF THE RISK OF NEURODEGENERATIVE DISEASES

Most of the diseases related to the aging of the brain take a long time to develop since the proteins present in and around the brain cells are misfolded, and they don't function like they are supposed to. As mentioned earlier, autophagy helps clean up all these malfunctioning proteins and reduces the accumulation of such proteins.

For instance, in Alzheimer's, autophagy removes amyloid, and in Parkinson's it removes α-synuclein. There is a reason why it is believed that dementia and diabetes go hand in hand with each other as constantly high levels of blood sugar prevent autophagy from kicking in, and this makes it quite difficult for cells to get rid of the clutter.

REGULATES INFLAMMATION

Do you remember the story of Goldilocks? How she found the perfect bed and the perfect bowl of porridge - that's not too hot or too cold, but just perfect? Likewise, autophagy helps regulate inflammation, and it produces a "Goldilocks" amount of inflammation in the body by either boosting or quelling the response of the immune system according to what your body needs.

Autophagy can increase the presence of inflammation by increasing it when there is an alien body in the body by triggering the defense mechanism of the immune system. Usually, autophagy decreases inflammation from the response of your immune system by getting rid of antigens that trigger it unnecessarily.

HELPS FIGHT INFECTIOUS DISEASES

As I have already mentioned, autophagy helps trigger the immune response as and when necessary. The autophagy mechanism helps get rid of specific microbes that are directly present within the cells like Mycobacterium tuberculosis or viruses like HIV. Autophagy also helps remove the toxins that are produced because of infections, especially any illness that's foodborne.

BETTER MUSCLE PERFORMANCE

Exercise results in slight microtears and slight inflammation of muscles, and this needs to be repaired. The demand for energy increases due to this. The cells in your muscles respond to this by inducing autophagy to reduce the energy that's necessary to use the muscle, eliminate the damaged bits and improve the overall balance of energy to decrease the risk of any future damage.

PREVENTS THE ONSET OF CANCER

Autophagy helps suppress the process that induces cancer like severe inflammation, instability in genomes, and the DNA response to damage. Studies on mice that have been genetically designed to suppress autophagy have shown an increased rate of cancer. As cancer progresses, it might activate autophagy to generate alternate fuel or to even hide from the immune system, but all the research so far has only been on animals and not on human beings.

BETTER DIGESTIVE HEALTH

The cells in the lining of the gastrointestinal tract are at work all the time. A large portion of your feces is cells. When autophagy is activated, your digestive cells have an opportunity to repair, restore, and clear themselves of any junk and reduce or trigger the immune system's reaction as needed.

Any chronic immune response in the gut can not only overwhelm your bowels, but it can also lead to inflammation within, so a chance to rest, repair and clean themselves is important for better digestive health. Autophagy gives your digestive system a much-needed respite from all the work it does.

BETTER SKIN HEALTH

The cells that are exposed in the body are vulnerable to a variety of damage from chemicals, air, light, humidity, pollution, and all forms of physical damage. It's quite a surprise that we don't look worse for wear given all that we expose our skin to. When your skin cells start to accumulate damage and toxins, then they begin to age.

Autophagy helps repair and replace these cells, and it makes your skin look fresh. Skin cells tend to engulf bacteria that can damage the body, so it is quintessential that you support them as they are clearing the clutter.

HEALTHY WEIGHT

Here are a couple of benefits of autophagy that help you maintain a healthy weight.

Short periods of fasting help activate autophagy, burn fat, hold on to muscle mass, and enable you to become lean and fit. It also reduces the chances of unnecessary inflammation that usually leads to weight gain. Autophagy helps reduce the levels of toxins in your body, and when this happens, the cells in your body will not retain a lot of fat.

Autophagy also supports your metabolic efficiency by repairing those parts of the cells that usually create and package proteins and synthesize energy, which is helpful when the cells need to start burning fat to provide energy.

REDUCES APOPTOSIS

Apoptosis is programmed cellular death. When compared to autophagy, apoptosis is quite messy, and it also creates more garbage that needs to be cleaned up. To assist in this cleanup, your body triggers inflammation. The more cells that are repaired, the less effort your body needs to make to clean away old cells and produce new ones.

Renewal of tissues requires less inflammation, so your body starts to use that energy to replace those cells that require constant renewal, like the cells in your digestive system or skin. While some cells need to be renewed regularly, there are some that don't. An increased effort to repair with fewer cleanups is a great combination for your body to function optimally.

CHAPTER 17: BENEFITS OF ONE MEAL A DAY

The popularity of intermittent fasting is increasing every day. One method of IF that is steadily becoming quite popular is the One Meal a Day diet, also known as the OMAD diet. Abstaining from food helps modulate your body's performance, and when you fast for prolonged periods, it has a positive effect on your body and mind.

The OMAD protocol is designed in such a manner that the fasting ratio you need to follow is 23:1. It means that your body will be effectively fasting for 23 hours, and the eating window is restricted to one hour. If you want to burn fat, trigger weight loss, improve your mental clarity, and reduce the time that you spend on food, then eating one meal a day is a brilliant idea.

The OMAD method oscillates between periods of eating and fasting. This method of fasting reduces the eating window more than the other diets. While following this dieting protocol, you need to make sure that you consume your daily calories within one meal and you fast for the rest of the day. OMAD helps you reap all the benefits of intermittent fasting, and it simplifies your schedule as well. The ideal time to break your fast is between 4 and 7 p.m. When you do this, you give your body sufficient time to start digesting the food that you eat before you sleep.

From the perspective of evolution, humans aren't designed to eat three meals per day. As mentioned earlier, our ancestor's bodies were used to functioning optimally even when there was food scarcity. Intermittent fasting protocols like the OMAD tend to kickstart various cell functions in your body that are helpful to improve your overall health. It can be quite intimidating to get started with this method of dieting. There are three simple tips that you can follow to make the transition easier on yourself.

The first thing that you need to do is *slowly cut back on the carbs* that you consume. If you want to optimize the results of this diet and want the least amount of crankiness, then you must limit your carb intake. When you consume a lot of carbs, your body tends to create a stock of glycogen in the body. If there is always some glucose present in your body, then your body will not be able to shift into ketosis. Ketosis is essential to kickstart the process of burning fats. So, if you are trying to start this diet, then it is a good idea to start by slowly cutting back on your carb intake.

You need to *ease your body into getting used to this fasting protocol*. It can be quite difficult to go from eating three meals a day to just one meal a day. You need to ease the transition so that it doesn't feel like you are suffering. A simple way in which you can do this is by slowly getting your body used to the idea of eating fewer meals. So, if you are used to eating three meals per day and tend to snack in between the meals, then the first step is to eliminate all the snacks. Then you can slowly increase the time between the meals and cut down on the number of meals you eat. If you do this, it will be quite easy to follow this diet.

Another simple way in which you can make this diet easier on your body is to consume some caffeine. A morning cup of coffee (devoid of milk and sugar) will make you feel fuller for longer and will keep your hunger pangs at bay.

KEY BENEFITS

WEIGHT LOSS

One of the primary benefits of intermittent fasting is weight loss. Intermittent fasting oscillates between periods of eating and fasting. While fasting, your calorie intake reduces naturally, and it helps you lose weight and maintain it as well. Apart from that, it also stops you from indulging in any form of mindless eating. Whenever you consume food, your body converts the food into glucose. The glucose that it needs immediately is converted into energy, and the rest is stored within the body in the form of fat cells. Not all the food you consume is converted into energy. So, all the unused energy is stored as fat within your cells. When you start to skip meals, your body will reach into its internal stores of energy. Once your body starts to burn fats to provide energy, it automatically starts the process of weight loss. Also, most of the fat is usually stored in the abdominal region. If you want to lose fat from your abdominal region, then this is the best diet for you.

SLEEP

Obesity is rampant these days. In fact, it is a major health problem that humanity is suffering from. The primary cause of obesity apart from terrible lifestyle and food choices is the lack of sleep. Intermittent fasting regulates your circadian rhythm, and encourages a better sleep cycle. When your body is sufficiently rested, it is capable of burning fats effectively. A good sleep cycle has several physiological benefits, like an increase in your energy levels and an overall improvement in your mood.

RESISTANCE TO ILLNESSES

Intermittent fasting assists in the growth as well as the regeneration of cells. Did you know that the human body has an internal mechanism for repairing all the damaged cells? Well, think of it as internal housekeeping that ensures that all the cells in your body are performing optimally. When you follow the protocols of intermittent fasting, it improves the overall functioning of your cells. So, it directly helps improve the natural defense mechanism in your body and increases the resistance to diseases as well as illnesses.

A HEALTHY HEART

Burning up all the stored unnecessary fats in the body helps improve your cardiovascular health. The buildup of plaque in the blood vessels is referred to as atherosclerosis. Atherosclerosis occurs when fat deposits start building up in the blood vessels, and it is the primary cause of different cardiovascular diseases. Endothelium is a thin lining present in the blood vessels, and a dysfunction of this lining causes atherosclerosis. Obesity is one of the main reasons for the build-up of plaque in blood vessels. Stress, as well as inflammation, worsens this problem. Intermittent fasting helps reduce and remove plaque deposits and helps tackle obesity. So, if you want to improve the health of your heart, then this is the best diet for you.

A HEALTHY GUT

Did you know that your gut is the home for several millions of microorganisms? These microorganisms are helpful and are essential for the optimal functioning of the digestive system. These microorganisms are known as microbiome. The gut microbiome is necessary for a healthy gut. A healthy digestive system helps with better absorption of food and improves the functioning of your stomach. So, a simple diet change can help you improve your gut's health.

TACKLES DIABETES

Diabetes is a terrible problem. In fact, it is right alongside with obesity as one of the leading health concerns these days. Diabetes is also a primary indicator for the risk of the increase of different cardiovascular diseases, like heart attacks and strokes. When the level of glucose is alarmingly high in the bloodstream, and there isn't sufficient insulin to process the glucose, it causes diabetes. When the body starts developing a resistance to insulin, it is quite difficult to regulate the sugar levels in the body. Intermittent fasting reduces the problem of insulin sensitivity and effectively helps tackle and manage diabetes.

REDUCES INFLAMMATION

Whenever your body notices an internal problem, it powers up its natural defense mechanism - inflammation. Inflammation in moderate amounts is desirable and helpful. However, it doesn't mean that all forms of inflammation are good. Excess inflammation causes various health problems like arthritics, atherosclerosis, and neurodegenerative disorders. Any inflammation of this form is known as chronic inflammation. Chronic inflammation is quite painful, and it can restrict your body's movements.

PROMOTES CELL REPAIR

When you start fasting, the cells in your body engage themselves in the process of waste removal. Waste removal refers to the process of breaking down dysfunctional cells and proteins. This process is known as autophagy and is quintessential for the upkeep of your body. Do you like accumulating waste in your home? Similarly, it is important to ensure that your body doesn't start collecting any toxic wastes. Autophagy is the natural way of getting rid of all unnecessary things from your body. Autophagy protects the neurons in your brain from any cell degeneration. It not only protects the neurons, but it also prevents them from excitotoxic stress. All this helps the brain replace the damaged cells and replace them with healthy new cells. When your body does this naturally, it improves the health of your brain. Autophagy also increases the lifespan of cells and promotes longevity.

IMPROVES MEMORY

Intermittent fasting also helps improve your ability to learn and retain things. Improving your memory is one of the best protective measures against neurodegenerative diseases. A diet that restricts the intake of calories helps improve your memory.

REDUCES DEPRESSION

Dealing with any mood disorder can be quite tricky. Medication isn't the only means to deal with such disorders. A healthy diet that doesn't fill your body with unnecessary calories leads to an overall improvement in mood. Not just mood, but it also improves your mental clarity and promotes alertness.

CHAPTER 18: FOODS THAT BOOST AUTOPHAGY

Following are some of the foods that stimulate autophagy:

GINGER

Ginger is a food that stimulates autophagy ghastly and makes things come close in an effective manner.

GREEN TEA

Green tea is the best drinking lot that can help you to be lean and adopt autophagy in you. It has some herbs and essential ingredients that are designed to give better illustrations to the people. The green tea is easy to mix and can be capitalized easily in the coming time. The green tea requires no such working in the products and can be available in every possible direction

REISHI MUSHROOMS

Reishi mushrooms can be easily accepted in the world timings, and these mushrooms could be made out of nowhere. The mushrooms make the body language more lenient in its desire, and with the passage of time, the people are able to learn a lot from its core and construct. The constructs of the mushrooms need to be identified with the passage of time, and they are best to carry out an autophagy product.

TURMERIC/CURCUMIN

Turmeric is a regimental disease that could be very healthy and compatible with autophagy. It does not require a lot of work for its process, and it could easily bring the concept of better regulations in the time. Therefore, the turmeric and curcumin are the best details looking forward to the people in the society.

Our bodies can detox themselves through natural processes in the livers, kidneys, skin, and bowels and through autophagy. However, we can also take special steps to detox ourselves through our diets and other lifestyle changes. This chapter is dedicated to the reasons why you might want to consider taking further steps to detox yourself.

Detox diets have earned a reputation of being based upon frivolous pseudoscience, but detoxing is an incredibly important process in our body. Our health is assaulted from all angles by toxins and pollutants, everything from caffeine and alcohol to air pollutants from industrial waste, car exhaust, and cigarette smoke. Most of the things we eat, even foods we consider healthy, have small amounts of toxic substances within them. Yet, we can also allow toxins to enter our bloodstream through the skin and through the air that enters our lungs. Regardless of their source, our body regularly needs to deal with all the nasty compounds and chemicals that end up in the body, otherwise, we can face corresponding nasty health consequences.

In the body, the liver and the kidneys are the organs responsible for dealing with toxins in the body. The kidneys filter toxins from the blood, whilst the liver breaks down toxins into substances that can be used by the body or passed without trouble. If the kidneys and liver are burdened with too many toxins or if they are not kept in good shape through a healthy lifestyle, they can be unable to deal with all the toxins in the body. This can cause a huge array of problems, anything from fatigue and general feelings of being unwell, to bloating and digestive problems and even liver disease.

Most detox diets are aimed at eating lots of foods that help keep the liver and kidney in tip-top shape, but there are also many other methods to keep these crucial organs healthy. Drinking lots of water – at least 6 to 8 glasses per day – allows any waste products of the liver and kidneys to easily pass through the body. Likewise, you should avoid smoking and second-hand cigarette smoke, which contains over 4,000 different chemicals, including 43 cancer-causing carcinogens.

Eating too much sugar also makes your liver unhappy. By now everyone knows how consuming too much sugar can contribute to diabetes and the various health issues associated with weight gain, but the effects of sugar on the liver remain an enigma to most. The liver has a very limited ability to metabolize sugar, with some dieticians suggesting that anything more than 6 teaspoons of added sugar is excessive. Any sugar that the liver cannot break down is stored as fat, and a build-up of fat in the liver can lead to a condition called fatty liver disease.

Fatty liver disease, in turn, can lead to more serious conditions as bodily pain, fatigue, weakness, and cirrhosis of the liver. Most people who are overweight or obese are at increased risk of fatty liver disease, and they may be suffering from the condition in its early stages when there are few explicit symptoms.

Caffeine is another common toxin that the body has to deal with regularly. Caffeine is commonly associated with coffee, but it is also present in most fizzy drinks, chocolate, and energy drinks. The liver interprets caffeine as a foreign chemical, and it is broken down through a special pathway in the liver that deals with manmade and unfamiliar substances, which includes most medication. For this reason, heavy caffeine consumption should especially be avoided when also taking certain drugs, especially pain relief chemicals such as acetaminophen.

Moderate caffeine consumption isn't dangerous or even unhealthy, with some studies suggesting it has numerous benefits on the body. Nonetheless, for the purposes of cleansing the body of toxins and giving the liver a period of relief, it's best to avoid this energy-booster or at least cut down on your silent addiction.

Good liver health can also be maintained by eating a diet rich in antioxidants, which aid in processing the waste products of toxins. Common antioxidants include vitamin C, vitamin E, beta-carotene, and zinc. Foods which are rich in antioxidants include dark chocolate, legumes, blueberries, red grapes, nuts, dark green veg, orange vegetable, and green tea.

You can also help detox through eating organic food whenever possible. Non-organic foods are free from pesticide residue that may be left on non-organic foods. Many pesticides can build up in the human body and may be dangerous in noticeable concentrations. Eating organic, however, isn't always possible, practical, or affordable, so sometimes it may be necessary to compromise. In general, if you eat the outer surface of grown food, it's more important that it is organic. Fruit such as strawberries, apples, grapes, cherries, and leafy greens should preferably be organic, whereas with fruit or veg with peel it is less important (such as bananas and onions). The easiest way to detox your body is always to avoid toxins in the first place!

There is also a detox method you might not expect; getting more sleep. The western world has an embarrassing relationship with sleep. Sleep is vital for our well-being in dozens of different ways – it's where we rest our minds and rejuvenate our body. Yet all too many people resent their need to sleep and try to cheat themselves out of an hour or two every night. This can take a serious toll on well-being.

In terms of detoxing and cleansing the body, most of the detox process occurs during sleep. In the resting state of sleep, your body is free to use resources and act in ways it simply can't when you are awake. For example, one of the main purposes of sleep is to filter toxins out of the brain, toxins which naturally as a side effect of being awake. The filtering system is called the lymphatic system, and it is thought to be 10 times more active during sleep than during wakefulness. During sleep, numerous other metabolic processes take part, such as those which occur in the liver and are inhibited whilst active.

Whilst it might be rather obvious, it is also worth mentioning that you can prevent toxins from getting into your system by avoiding places and environments where there are toxins present. Exhaust fumes, second-hand smoke, and low air quality from industrial pollution are the main culprits, but depending on your location and career you may come into contact with many other types of toxins such as chemical residue from working in a factory, for example.

You can also aid the detox process by taking certain supplements, most notably milk thistle. Milk thistle is a small plant that grows in Mediterranean regions. It can be used as a herb, and it also goes by the names Mary Thistle or Holy Thistle. Milk thistle is a popular natural choice for helping treat liver conditions such as cirrhosis or jaundice, and it is also a staple of the detox community.

The active ingredient in milk thistle is called silymarin, and it has powerful anti-inflammatory properties as well as being an anti-oxidant. Research on silymarin is still progressing, and it's not entirely clear how it affects the body. Some studies have suggested that silymarin can aid liver function in individuals who have been exposed to industrial toxins, such as xylene, and there is evidence to help it also improves type 2 diabetes and lowers cholesterol.

Finally, you can also try a temporary cleansing diet. Ultimately, our body needs the right materials to detox, and as you might now understand, our regular diets don't give us enough resources to work with. You can rectify this by trying a cleansing diet intended to give your body a huge boost of all the vitamins, minerals, and good stuff it needs to cleanse itself.

Of course, ideally, a healthy, balanced diet will help the body cleanse itself over time and be exposed to fewer toxins. However, whether it's due to personal fault or factors beyond our control, we can't always consume a perfectly healthy diet. It might just be too pricey, we might not have the time, or we might constantly be around other people who influence or control our eating habits.

Therefore, as a temporary solution or as a compromise, you can periodically embrace a cleansing detox diet. These types of diets aren't intended to be a permanent change to your eating patterns, and you shouldn't follow them for any period longer than 1-week. However, with that being said, they can give your body a reprieve to repair and rejuvenate itself, a benefit that can last for a few weeks or months before being required once more.

There are many different types of cleansing and detox diets, most of which involve consuming a large amount of fruit, vegetables, and calorie-free drinks. Try one out for a week and see how you feel afterward!

EAT PROBIOTICS!

If you decide to detox, it might seem like the list of prohibited foods is huge. However, there are still many great choices for a detox diet, and you should still find that you can eat a diverse and tasty diet during your detox and body cleanse.

In particular, *probiotics* are a good choice. Probiotics are a group of foods that contain 'good' bacteria that promote a healthy gastrointestinal ecosystem. As you may know, your gut contains tens of thousands of different bacteria, some of which can benefit your health, some which cause harm, and some which have little impact. The health of the bowels is increasingly understood to be crucial to human health, with some studies suggesting that the flora of the gut influencing how many nutrients and calories you absorb from your food and even contributing to mood swings and depressions. In fact, probiotics have also been argued to help prevent diarrhea, gut disease and improve eczema, although the support for these claims is controversial.

There are many different probiotic foods, including yogurt, sauerkraut, miso soup, kefir, sourdough bread, and tempeh, all of which are considered healthy detox-friendly foods, at least when eaten in moderation. Probiotics can also be found as a supplement, although if you decide to take a specific probiotic supplement it's worth further researching what the proposed benefits are – there are many different types of probiotic supplement all of the different supposed effects.

CHANGING YOUR EATING HABITS

Whether you are attempting a detox diet or trying to fast, you are not only working against your natural instinct to eat, but any habits and emotions that revolve around food. You might eat when you are tired to give you a boost in energy, binge to perk up your mood, or make poor choices just out of routine or mindlessness. Regardless of your reasons for a detox diet or a fast to work, you need to control how you interact with food.

Start by thinking about your current habits. Are you an emotional eater? Do you like to reward yourself with food? The first stage to overcoming these habits is simply recognizing them and being honest with yourself. It's better to admit your faults rather than to pretend that they don't exist; they'll be there regardless.

By acknowledging how you interact with food you can anticipate and prepare for any temptations that occur during your fast or detox. By depriving yourself of food or by forcing yourself to eat a cleansing diet, you will encounter these feelings, and they will probably be stronger than they usually are.

Learn to challenge your feelings and your thoughts. Are you really hungry? Do you really need to give up on your fast? Isn't there an alternate more productive way to deal with your emotions? Try meditating or doing some activity, such as walking your dog or tackling a task you've been putting off. By engaging with an activity you consider positive you'll feel much better afterward, and the emotions that were bothering you will dissipate.

Also, learn to just sit and be comfortable with your feelings. Instead of shying away from the emotional pain that might be driving you to binge eat, or simply the lack of motivation to continue, take a moment to pause in your day and explore these feelings. Are they strong or weak? How do they affect your thought patterns? How are these feelings affecting your body – can you explore where these feelings are actually occurring? The more you learn to delve into these feelings instead of running away, the more mundane they will become and the less influence they will have over you.

You should also make an effort to be mindful of your eating patterns, in both a detox diet and an eating pattern that involves fasting. You might find that you gorge on your food without truly considering or tasting it, or when you come home from work you automatically start browsing around in the fridge for something to snack on. By trying to be more aware of your interactions with food, you can help manage temptations and habits that urge you to eat.

Finally, try to think positively about your detox diet or fast. Studies have shown that it's easier to change your habits by developing positive habits rather than breaking negative habits. Or in other words, instead of thinking 'I want to stop feeling so lethargic and bloating, it's better to think 'I want to be successful in my detox diet.' These two thoughts might relate to the same goal, but the latter has a much more positive vibe to it, which also makes it easier to strive towards.

DEALING WITH OTHER PEOPLE

Many people won't appreciate the benefits of fasting or a detox diet. You can cite a hundred different studies or try to explain your motivations as logically and clearly as possible, but people might still sneer or disregard what you are doing.

As a result, it's best to consider carefully who you talk about your diet. Do they need to know? Does it bother you if you don't have their approval? It might not be a big deal if someone doesn't accept your diet, but it can still make your life easier if you are not listening to snide comments or objections every time you are around them.

You can always find support online or a detox and fasting community nearby to talk to. These people will understand you and be more welcoming. Of course, you may be fortunate to be surrounded by friends and family who are considerate, or at the very least, appreciate what you are doing is important to you.

If you have to tell people, just try and be as clear and reasonable about the discussion as possible. Laying a strong foundation for why you are doing a fast or detox diet will help people accept it; if your first explanation is watertight, people will find it hard to object, yet if you explain yourself poorly, you'll be dogged by criticism throughout.

CHAPTER 19: CIRCADIAN RHYTHMS AND AUTOPHAGY

Whether you're a night owl or an early bird, getting a good night of sleep goes beyond just improving your mood. Sleep has implications in nearly every system in the body: it boosts cardiovascular health, helps to lose weight, improves your memory, lower stress levels, and is crucial to help the immune system battle infections. During the night, the body goes into "repair mode" and starts cleaning the damage done to the cells during the day, especially in the nervous system. (*Altun, A. and Ugur-Altun, B. 2007; Xie, L. et al. 2013*)

Neurons in the brain oversee all functions in the body, firing electrical impulses, ordering hormone release to regulate your metabolism, and processing external stimuli. This extreme cellular activity causes metabolites and toxins to accumulate inside neurons, namely adenosine, a molecular byproduct of ATP degradation. When adenosine levels rise in the brain, the neuronal function can be impaired. In fact, many neurodegenerative diseases - like Alzheimer's and Lewy body dementia – as well as psychiatric and mood disorders can be linked with poor sleep. (*He, Y. et al. 2016; Ma, D. et al. 2012*)

Sounds familiar? A decrease in autophagy levels is also associated with neuropathies, where astrocytes are unable to remove and degrade accumulated proteins in their lysosomes and avoid neuron destruction, and there are reports that link sleep and autophagy as essential processes for tissue housekeeping and metabolic regulation. In 1970, a series of microscopy studies pointed out that the number of autophagosomes in mice cardiomyocytes, hepatocytes, pancreatic and renal cells varied throughout the day, in a similar fashion to the circadian rhythm. (*Ma, D. et al. 2012*)

In mammals, sleep and metabolism are regulated by the suprachiasmatic nucleus (SNC), which is responsible for establishing the circadian rhythm, a 24-hour cycle in which many biological parameters – from blood sugar levels, hormonal concentrations, to feeding signals – vary in distinct diurnal patterns and are prevalent in tissues with high metabolic activity.

At the same time, gene expression in the liver, SCN, and other tissues involved in metabolism also vary, especially for genes that participate in glucose and lipid metabolism. Bmal-1 and Rev-erbα expression, in particular, was significantly increased, and was later found that it happens along with a peak in autophagic flux. Bmal-1 knock-out mice were diagnosed with an impairment in gluconeogenesis and hypoglycemia, that increased at night, resulting from an impairment in autophagy.

Cyclic activation of autophagy and its respective regulation genes is therefore considered to be a cellular response to changes in metabolic gears, and if it stops functioning correctly, it can increase the risk of many diseases that were already described. For example, mice that were engineered to express symptoms of Alzheimer's disease showed a cyclic pattern of beta-amyloid protein aggregation, based on how fragmented their sleep cycle was. Autophagy cycles were particularly altered in the hippocampus, the first structure to be affected by a lack of sleep – often leading to memory loss. (*Maiese, K., 2017; Hastings, M. and Goedert, M. 2013*)

Additionally, melatonin levels were altered in mice with sleep deficits, affecting how mTOR regulation of aging and neurodegeneration occurred. Melatonin is the main hormone to regulate sleep cycles and can be severely repressed if we don't keep a regular sleep schedule. (*Merenlender-Wagner, A. et al. 2013*)

CHAPTER 20: SLEEP OPTIMIZATION

Modern society promotes a lifestyle that does not allow for normal circadian rhythms. The use of alarms to wake us up before a shift, artificial lights at our homes that prolong the daylight period in circadian cycles, and using electronic devices before going to sleep are factors that greatly influence our sleep cycles. Endogenously, our melatonin levels are regulated by light/darkness levels, and exposure to longer cycles contributes to a dramatic shift in its production.

Observational studies with populations of the Amazon jungle have confirmed these suspicions. These populations had no access to electric light, and their sleep cycles were longer by 30 minutes than occidental populations. This phenomenon is becoming even more common in an increasingly technological, nocturnal, and competitive world, a byproduct of our working schedules.

This hypothesis takes particular relevance in countries that have flourished technologically in the post-war, as in the case of South Korea and Japan. South Korea is highly competitive in academic and work terms, where sleep time is shortened when economic circumstances so dictate, being inversely correlated with time spent at work and salary.

However, these trends have mixed standards in many countries, with varying literature within the same country. These contradictory data do not, in any way, refuse the idea that chronic sleep deprivation has a high prevalence in adults. Any adult aged 25 to 64 years old requires on average 7 to 9 hours of sleep per day, but, according to the CDC, about 34.8% of American adults sleep less than 7 hours a day and have a clearly deficient sleep time with cumulative negative effects. In addition to this, there has been a decline in the sleep hours that children and adolescents get in the past decades. Dollman et al. verified a decrease of about 30 minutes in their daily sleep schedules between 1985 and 2004 in Australian children aged 10 to 15 years. This pattern has been identified in other nations such as Japan, Switzerland, and Iceland. These findings may have some clinical relevance in the appearance of certain pathologies such as hyperactivity disorder with deficit attention, as some differences were observed across studies with children living with this pathology – mainly a shorter sleep duration, increased latency period, patterns of movement during sleep - relative to healthy children.

It is known that most of these changes affect people at an endocrinological level, especially when they only a few hours of sleep per day. Serum levels of cortisol and ghrelin rise and make a considerable increase in appetite and the risk for diabetes or obesity, cardiovascular diseases. There are also consequences for the immune system, where people that sleep less than 6 hours a day can have a decrease or increase in immunological activity, meaning that they are more sensitive to infectious diseases.

Problems related to sleep are also an additional risk factor for accidents at work and for road accidents. To this end, in attention, concentration, increased reaction time, distraction, stress, and irritability. In 2003, a study involving more than 7000 workers from several Dutch industries showed that workers with high rates of fatigue were 70% more likely to be involved in work-related accidents, compared with workers reporting low levels of fatigue, with many of these accidents resulting in fatalities.

If we dive deeper into this knowledge, we can see that biological rhythms exist in all living organisms and regulate many functions, from physiological and mental processes. The grouping of these patterns make up our chronotype, or our individual preference to rest during the day. The disruption of these rhythms is one of the aspects present in depressive syndromes, with many documented setbacks in patients with major depressive disorders, bipolar disorders, and seasonal affective disorders.

In recent decades, a new line of thinking linked the appearance of these disorders with deregulation in autophagy, and that just like we're used to taking the trash out late at night, cells initiate their clean up process at specific times of the day. For example, researchers have found that mice expressing Alzheimer's disease and were sleep deprived for a few days showed higher levels of beta-amyloid, a protein that accumulates in the brain of patients diagnosed with this disease. One of the structures that were more affected by a change in sleep cycles was the hippocampus, which is a tiny bean on our brain that helps us remember facts and things that happen to us during the day. Neurons inside the hippocampus had difficulties starting autophagy, and this sudden block made them less capable to fight back the formation of beta-amyloid.

In any cell, autophagy happens like a dance, in a rhythmic manner, and this dance is choreographed not only by sleep cycles. Metabolism and sleep go hand in hand when it comes to regulating our biological clock. Some metabolic syndromes are caused by terrible sleeping habits, leading to weight gain, hormonal diseases, and cardiovascular diseases. This happens because there are genes that are extremely sensitive to these changes, and they happen to be associated with metabolic processes. Screening of liver, neuronal, and muscular tissues showed that their genetic expression varies according to the time of day and sugar levels, with bmal-1 and Rev-erbα being the most altered in their expression. Surprisingly, so did autophagy levels.

As researchers dived further into this rabbit hole, they found that mice with low Bmal-1 levels had more chances of becoming hypoglycemic during the day, and why? Because they couldn't activate autophagy. It was a breakthrough when they found that there was a cycle behind this process and that autophagy was present in higher levels after the mice were fed and lowered at night before they went to rest. The same happens to us. Ever wondered why you feel extremely tired at night? That's your circadian clock working and signaling your body to rest and digest: you are fed, and you are ready to start repairing your body with a good night's sleep. Autophagy is shut down at this time as stress levels go down.

But wait, isn't autophagy supposed to help us repair our bodies? Of course, but autophagy is not a major regeneration mechanism when we sleep. Autophagy is like insurance we have on our cells during the day, that helps them fight back all the damage and stress they take. Nevertheless, it is important to have a good night's sleep, as not to disrupt your autophagic cycles. If you are having trouble keeping your eyes shut at night, don't lose sleep over it, and check out the tips below to have a healthy sleep cycle.

CONCLUSION

To conclude the book, you have to be very careful about the diet intakes that you do throughout your routine. You need to be curious about every calorie that goes into you. You have been provided with all the reasons in this book about the process of autophagy. Autophagy can give you a healthy ph and can avert any harmful stroke of acidity in the body. Acidity can be dangerous in profuse accumulation of fats, rise to inflammatory disease, the rupture in many digestion organs, and having a rusted metabolism that does not work in the flow. On the contrary, autophagy can give you a fresh intake of all healthy diets that can be very healthy and caring for you. These diets are present in all formats.

They are in breakfast recipes, the dinner recipes, the lunch recipes, the smoothies, and the sweat desserts that can up-satisfaction in your mouth. You do not have to be an expert in medicine to know which diet to follow when. You just have to know the diet intake of your own body and see how you are able to cater to the plight of diseases. You must not be able to compound yourself with the attack of acidity, but must have the courage to use these diets and recover at the earliest.

These diets have everything in their DNA. They have the minerals, the enzymes, the protein, the amino acids, and whatnot. Green refluxes along with curing liquids are present in these diets, and they come in all whims and fancies of the diet expression. There is no rocket science behind their creation, and one has to be very intelligent while creating them. You can also follow this book and will get a splendid amount of results in no time. It is available at an affordable price.

Try your best to avoid any acidic diet at all costs, even if it gives you a great amount of relish. The idea is fats and minerals are very delicious, but they come with devious outcomes of fat accumulation and strengths. You need to understand that long aging is only possible if you have a balanced diet intake, and this diet can be only an alkaline one.

To make conclusive remarks of the book about the benefits of an alkaline diet, first and foremost is the sheer activeness that a person tends to achieve while he is eating an alkaline diet. He feels healthy and looks healthy and wants to be doing a lot of things while he has an alkaline diet. He can think properly and can get rid of inflammatory diseases that can cause him suffering. He has a strong discipline that can be navigated in any way possible, and thus, he is the next big thing for his users. Also, the longevity of life in this scenario and truly, autophagy can do a lot of wonders for the individual. Therefore, autophagy has a lot to do with the fitness and active-ness in the human body.

Furthermore, If you want to look green and fresh on your face, then autophagy can be very helpful in this regard. Studies show that autophagy is very popular in making a healthy face for you. The number of herbs and breakfast recipes you have for yourself up-bring a good amount of freshness on your face as well on your skin. Thus, autophagy is very crucial for having great skin and face.

You are able to get a lot of chronic pains in your body due to many reasons. You get to the bottom of any problem; you solve it and end up having chronic pain in your body. Chronic pain refers to any tertiary amount of pain in your body, and you are able to get to the harmfulness of it in no time. Therefore, chronic pain is the most devastating headache that you can get, and the only effective cure for it is the alkaline diet. Yes, autophagy is very important for you to maintain as the blood level minimizes when lemon or other alkaline water is induced in the body. So, this is another benefit of autophagy, and it does not matter if you are a walker, a boxer, or even a corporate worker, you must have autophagy in you if you wish to give all that you crave.

In the end, we will only assure you good health and being a beginner, you must waste any further time and order this book in a jiffy. Because health is wealth, nobody became rich while being lazy and stubborn. This book is all that you need, and you must get at all costs.

CPSIA information can be obtained
at www.ICGtesting.com
Printed in the USA
LVHW050938210221
679536LV00034B/1197